SOCIAL ALCOHOL

Is It *Really* a Good Drug?

Dale B. Sherrod, M.D.

A Collection of Essays

ISBN-13: 978-1978441866
ISBN-10: 197844186X

Dedicated to
Humanity

Acknowledgements

I want to thank my family for their great support as work
has progressed on this book. My children and their spouses
Ray and Kitty Sherrod, Gwen and Guerin Green, Susan
and Andy Lillie and their tremendous children,
have supported me all the way.

My three friends Paul Flanders, Jeff Linroth and
Tim Jolly have spurred me onward,
not allowing me to loaf or waste time.
Linda Veach has been a great help.

Editing this book has not been simple
and for that, I thank
John and Darlene Chilson.

Any errors of spelling, punctuation,
grammar, theology or anything else
are purely mine and, when found, will
be corrected in a future edition.

Chapters

Preface

This book is designed for everyone from age 10 to age 90 and beyond. I hope that elementary school students will enjoy it, as well as people with advanced college educations, perhaps with several college degrees.

All of my adult life, I have been an MD, seeing patients in private practice, in the US Army Medical Corps and I have served on the faculty at the University of Colorado School of Medicine. In our country, doctors do good jobs of screening for and making great efforts to prevent, many potentially fatal cancers, such as cancers of the breast, cervix and prostate.

Despite vigorous and very expensive screening techniques, these three cancers still have death rates of 42,000 per year for breast cancer, 6,000 per year for cervical cancer, and 27,000 per year for prostate cancer. [1]

If we total the deaths of the above three mentioned cancers which are vigorously screened for, we get 75,000 deaths per year, despite intensive screening. If we compare those 75,000 cancer deaths to deaths from alcohol, we find that alcohol kills 88,000 Americans, men, women and children, per year [2]*, although some experts say that alcohol kills more than 100,000 people per year. [3] Beyond alcohol's death rate, we have many types of morbidly from that drug, including permanent injury, paralysis, loss of limbs and more.

* This 88,000 annual alcohol related deaths is from the U.S. Center for Disease Control in their Bulletin, May 2017. It will be quoted more than once in various chapters but the reference [2] will not be shown each time.

Social Alcohol

Like many doctors who want to stay current, I have, in my training, attended dozens of courses, classes, seminars and educational sessions regarding the prevention of cancer. In fact, we MDs are bombarded with ads and information about excellent courses to attend on cancer prevention. But I cannot remember receiving any type of notice or ad mentioning how doctors can prevent the 88,000 yearly deaths from alcohol. I do not recall one class in four years of medical school which addressed prevention of the 88,000 yearly alcohol deaths.

Hence, the subject of this book. Why do we doctors focus our skills on certain killers and not on others?

This book focuses only on the United States; other countries are not addressed. All statistics relate only to the United States unless otherwise noted.

My good friend, Chip Haring, was killed in a car–truck accident. Before his death, he and I had many tremendous discussions. One of his favorite comments was that if he had a strong idea and if he vocalized it, he was delighted if someone could prove him wrong. That is my approach to this book.

Please email me if you have ideas, pro or con. Your comments are welcome. I'll do my best to answer. My email address is available on the outside of the back cover of this book.

Dale Sherrod, MD

Introduction

Some Doctors Are Speaking Out

A short time before this book went to press, I discovered a policy statement by a large group of physicians who treat cancer — the American Society of Clinical Oncologists (ASCO) with a membership of over 44,000 oncology professionals. [4]

Their policy statement was originally published in the Lancet, one of the most prestigious medical journals in the world. [5] It was then reprinted in the Journal of Clinical Oncology and included the facts that the drinking of alcohol is an established risk factor for several malignancies (cancerous growths).

Alcohol use is firmly associated with cancer of the larynx (voice box), throat cancer, cancer of the esophagus, liver cancer, breast cancer and colon cancer. Even modest alcohol use increases these risks, but the greatest risks occur with heavy, prolonged, alcohol use.

In their policy statement, Bruce Johnson, M.D., the president of ASCO, stated that people in the USA do not typically associate beer, wine, and hard liquor with an increased risk for cancer, but the relation is firmly established. Consequently, ASCO supports New York City's ban on alcohol ads on city buses and in subways.

Also, ASCO supports the elimination of "pinkwashing," a ploy to market alcoholic beverages by exploiting the color pink or pink ribbons.

Social Alcohol

"Pinkwashing" is a movement by the alcohol industry to display pink ribbons at sporting events. They also often place pink ribbon stickers on bottles of alcohol, suggesting to women the alcohol industry is concerned about breast cancer. Of course, alcohol consumption is proven to increase female breast cancer. [4]

The alcohol industry wants to show to the public their "commitment" to finding a cure for breast cancer. This is strange given the evidence that alcohol consumption is linked to the increased risk of breast cancer.

Elsewhere in this book, I discuss how pink ribbons are sometimes placed on the football fields of the National Football League (NFL). *This occurs even though the NFL provides no money for breast cancer treatment or research.* *

In 2017 the NFL made a change in its rules which eliminated the prior ban of hard liquor ads on TV. For the first—time whiskey, vodka, rum and other spirits are allowed to advertise during NFL games. [6]

Do you see irony here?

The NFL ...

- ✓ places pink ribbons on football fields
- ✓ increases their ads for alcohol use
- ✓ wants the public to be aware of the NFL's concern about breast cancer, which is increased with more alcohol use
- ✓ while the NFL provides no funds for breast cancer prevention or treatment.

** See Page 25 — NFL, Breast Cancer Awareness and Alcohol Awareness*

Definitions

Alcohol: A colorless liquid that is the intoxicating constituent of wine, beer, spirits and other drinks.

Alcoholism: A condition, often progressive and fatal, which involves lack of control of drinking alcohol. *

Alcohol Use Disorder (AUD): Synonymous with alcoholism. *

Mortality: Death rate resulting from any activity.

Morbidity: Serious reduction of physical, mental, or social activity as a result of any activity. For example, skydiving could have a high morbidity rate due to fractured limbs. Or alcohol can have a high morbidity rate, when an inebriated person has a car crash, resulting in permanent paralysis of a car passenger.

See page 146 for more detailed definitions.

1
Rationalization

Any human may use any type of rationalization to prove any point relating to alcohol use in themselves or others.

Rationalization on this subject can be universal.

2

Anyone Can Be Convinced of Anything

Respected and experienced politicians, in dealing with world affairs, have stated that, given the right circumstance, any country can be convinced about anything. Also, politicians have stated, given the right circumstance, any person can be convinced about anything. Of course, these statements may not be true, obviously.

But consider these statements, when applied to social alcohol. Given the right circumstances, about any person can be convinced that social alcohol, destructive as it is, can be the right thing. It can be stylish, it may taste OK and it can make people feel good temporarily.

The chore of convincing someone to drink social alcohol is not difficult to do.

3

I Know What I Believe and I Know I Am Right

There is a human tendency present, probably, in many of us, about any subject, to come to a conclusion about a situation.

This human tendency includes the fact that a human gets information and, after obtaining a conclusion, states to himself/herself and to the world, "Here's what I believe, and I feel that I am right."

This tendency occurs in politics, theology, race relations and in many other aspects of our lives. This tendency is certainly prevalent regarding the subject of alcohol.

For example, total abstainers feel that they are correct. Individuals who drink one glass of wine daily feel they are right. People who use eight ounces of distilled spirits per day may feel their way is correct.

Folks who drink eight beers per day may feel their way is correct. This tendency to "know that I am right" is not present in all humans, but it is a common tendency.

This tendency is often present on the subject of alcohol. It is easy for an individual to encounter the subject of alcohol, come to a conclusion about whether he/she will/will not use it and to defend this as the correct approach.

In this book, I am striving for objectivity and the minute that I say that, I realize that it is very difficult to maintain complete objectivity on sensitive subjects. The subject of alcohol is packed with facts, experiences, anecdotes, emotions and opinions.

Also, the subject is politically and financially packed. The alcohol industry spends large amounts of money on lobbying designed to convince members of the U.S. Congress to support the alcohol industry.

4
Statistics

Do we think that statistics are boring? The following are not.

- ✓ In the USA, 51% of adults age 18 and over are regular drinkers. [7]
- ✓ 12.4% of U S men are alcoholics, while 4.9% of women are alcoholics. [8]
- ✓ Look at any group of 100 men —
  ### *12 are alcoholics.*
- ✓ Look at any group of 100 women —
  ### *5 are alcoholics.*

These numbers are staggering.

These statistics are not boring. They are tragic.

5

That's the Way We've Always Done It

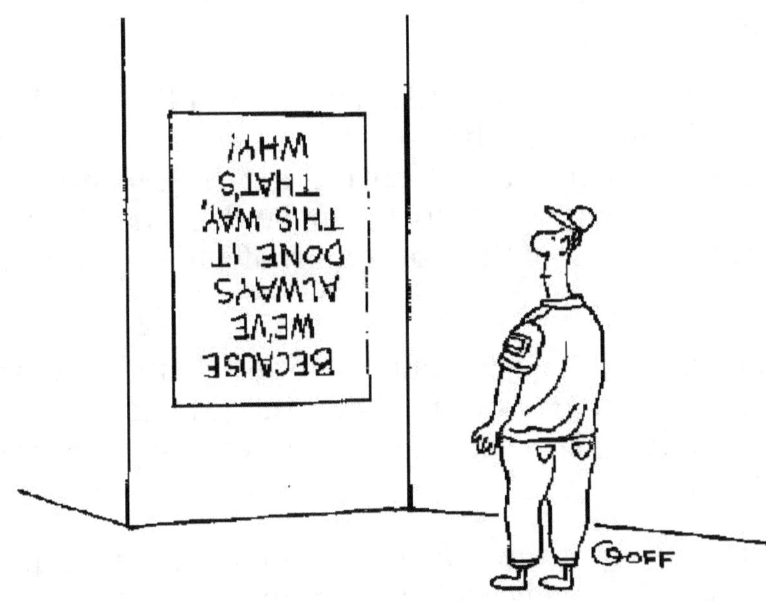

6

Strong Advice from WHO and Governments

A recent publication by Chaudhuri [9] had a good summary of America's current approach to alcohol. The review states that for several years, beer, wine and liquor producers have been pleased by a theory, proposed in the early 1970s by Klatsky [10], that a small amount of daily alcohol could provide modest heart and other health benefits.

But in recent years, scientists from around the world have been shifting their thoughts away from the potential benefits of alcohol and focusing on the cancer risks of alcohol. In January of 2016, England changed its prior advice that had said that some daily alcohol could help the heart.

England issued new guidelines, noting that alcohol raises the risk of certain cancers. The Chief Medical Officer of England, Sally Davies, stated, "There is no safe level of drinking." [9]

A study group from the government of Great Britain concluded, "There is no justification for drinking alcohol for health reasons." [11]

In America, the U.S. Department of Health and Human Services deleted their older suggestion that small amounts of drinking might decrease the risk of heart problems for some people. Currently, in the U S Government's Dietary Guidelines [12], there is no mention of health benefits of alcohol.

Strong Advice from WHO and Governments

The World Health Organization (WHO) in 2017 [7] stated that there is *no safe level* (italics by author) for drinking alcohol.

Despite the hard, solid evidence from respected scientists, some consumer publications can still be found stating, "A little daily alcohol may be good for you."

In England, scientists stated that alcohol in any amount is associated with a higher incidence of breast cancer, mouth cancer, throat cancer and other types of cancer.

In the USA, Dr. Anne McTiernan reported extensive research on the relation between alcohol and breast cancer. She reported that even one drink per day causes a 5% increase in breast cancer in premenopausal women and the same amount of daily alcohol causes a 9% increase in breast cancer in postmenopausal women. [13]

Scientific personalities may get involved, since whether to drink or to not drink is very important to the alcohol industries worldwide. In Boston, Dr. Tim Naimi does research on alcohol, obtaining funding from government grants. Dr. Curtis Ellison, also in Boston, does alcohol research, having obtained funding from the alcohol industry.

(In scientific research, it is common for industries to pay researchers grant money, hoping that the results will be favorable to their industries, not just in the field of alcohol.)

Social Alcohol

Dr. Naimi found major flaws in Klatsky's earlier research indicating that alcohol might help the heart and Dr. Naimi's conclusion was that alcohol had zero health benefits. Dr. Ellison, in the same Boston building as Dr. Naimi, criticized Dr. Naimi's research methods.

These two well informed doctors had a vigorous public debate in 2014, greatly disagreeing on the "bad" versus the "good" effects of alcohol on humans. From my viewpoint, I feel that Dr. Ellison, who has obtained funding from the alcohol industry, is incorrect. I feel that Dr. Naimi is correct, when he states that alcohol has zero health benefits. Dr. Naimi has never received funding from alcohol industries.

In summary, Dr. Klatsky's advice from the early 70s that a small amount of daily alcohol could help the heart, is being overshadowed by more modern research, which states that there is no health benefit from alcohol, which has definite risks and dangers. [14] [15] [16] [17] [18] [19] [20] [21] [22]

(Since Dr. Ellison has received funding from the alcohol industry, I am discounting his opinion that alcohol has some health benefits. I agree with the World Health Organization, British scientists and American scientists; as well as the British government and the US Government, that there are no health benefits from alcohol.)

This entire discussion on whether small amounts of alcohol help or do not help the heart, is somewhat like a novel or a drama which started in 1974. Here is what happened:

Strong Advice from WHO and Governments

In 1974, Dr. Klatsky published a report indicating that small amount of alcohol might prevent later heart trouble. This research was hailed as new information that might help many people. This first report by Klatsky was not funded by the alcohol industry. But the alcohol industry approved of his 1974 findings, and the alcohol industry paid Klatsky to do future research projects, which they hoped would add credibility to his original 1974 report.

News media and advertisers picked up on the 1974 project, and many lay publications, as well as ads, mentioned the alleged heart advantages of small amounts of daily alcohol. But, soon after the 1974 report, scientists who were not funded by the alcohol industry, started asking questions about Klatsky's methods and conclusions.

Many of these scientists found his original methods faulty and his 1974 conclusions not valid. Numerous papers were published in medical journals, stating that Klatsky's 1974 conclusions were not valid. [22] [21] [20] [19] [18] [17] [23] [16] [24] [15] [25] [14] [26]

Even Dr. Klatsky, in 2015, made the honest and courageous statement that "The apparent benefits of light to moderate alcohol consumption on the heart are controversial." [27] He was striving for objectivity, and the scientific community applauded his frankness.

In the meantime, the alcohol industry has not given up. Dr. Curtis Ellison, who received research funding from the alcohol industry and who championed the possible heart protective benefits of alcohol, joined with the International Center for Alcohol Policies (ICAP), a non–profit group supported by the alcohol industry, to host a large conference on the subject.

Social Alcohol

This conference was partially funded by the alcohol industry. The summary of the conference was written by Dr. Ellison and by Marjana Martinic, a senior vice president of ICAP which paid for printing and distribution of tens of thousands of copies of the conference summary.

These copies were included as free inserts in two popular medical journals, *The American Journal of Medicine* and the *American Journal of Cardiology*. Busy medical doctors then saw these inserts, which encouraged the false notion of the alleged heart protective benefits of alcohol. [23]

The drama continues: Since then many scientists and researchers have published articles in medical journals showing evidence that alcohol does not protect against heart trouble. Some examples include:

✓ Naimi, et al, published a paper stating that "prior studies about health effects of drinking should be interpreted with great caution." [22]

✓ Roerecke, "A heart protective association of alcohol cannot be assumed." [26]

✓ Chikritchs, et al, published an article with the title: "A healthy dose of skepticism: Good reasons to think again about the protective effects of alcohol in the heart." The conclusion of the article was: "The strength of evidence for protective effect of alcohol on the heart could be misguided. Few studies have correctly addressed the issue." [14]

✓ Zhao, et al, stated that "we cannot conclude that alcohol causes a decrease in heart disease." [20]

✓ Fillmore, et al, "Errors may be operating in former research showing protection of alcohol against heart disease." [16]

✓ Andreasson, et al, "There are reasons for skepticism about evidence that alcohol consumption can protect the heart." [18]

✓ Knott, et al, "The protective effect of alcohol on heart health may be explained by faulty research methods of Klatsky, including selection bias." [17]

✓ Daube, "Alcohol has evaporating health benefits. Alcohol industry promotion and lobbying are rife and unchecked by governments. Given the harms attributed to alcohol use, it is not surprising that the older reports suggesting benefits from low level alcohol use attracted enthusiasm among consumers, the media, and the alcohol industry.

> "These apparent benefits are now evaporating, born out by recent research. If there is any beneficial dose–response relation, it is limited to women aged 65 or more and even that association is at best modest and likely to be explained by selection bias." [19]

From the early days in the 1970's, headlines such as "a few drinks a day may help curb heart attacks" promoted messages about the beneficial effects of drinking. Many well–meaning doctors felt comfortable advising patients that alcohol consumption could be beneficial, and politicians used evidence on possible benefits to justify their failure to act on reducing harms.

As this book's author and as a reader of medical literature, I have noted that reports showing the invalidity of Katsky's original 1974 research have been coming out for ten or more years. That is why the World Health Organization, the British government, and others have stated that there are no health benefits from alcohol.

Social Alcohol

So, I was puzzled when, upon reading the March 2016 issue of the *Mayo Clinic Health Letter* [28], there was still the suggestion that low to moderate alcohol intake could be beneficial to the heart.

I contacted the managing editor of the *Mayo Clinic Health Letter*, wondering why their publication was still printing the invalid, older advice. He stated that the board of directors of his publication were studying the subject. His reply puzzled me, and I am uncertain about why he answered in that way.

Sometime soon I plan to embark on the labor–intensive task of identifying all the names on their board of directors to determine if any of them are doing research funded by the alcohol industry or have connections to the alcohol industry.

7

Black Diamond Routes

In Annie Grace's book, "This Naked Mind," [29] she discusses reasons people drink and mentions the "Black Diamond Effect."

That is, when a family is skiing, some adult mentions that he or she will do some skiing on a Black Diamond route. These routes are very difficult and, possibly, dangerous. The child asks if he or she can join the adult, who mentions that the child is not old enough and must wait until later in life when more skiing skills have developed. Only then will the child be old enough to enjoy Black Diamond routes.

Grace mentions that this ski analogy may apply when an adult tells a young person, "You must wait until you are older before you use alcohol." This phenomenon defines a prize which a child may look forward to later in life — a prize like obtaining a driver's license or obtaining other rites of passage.

Before the legal age of drinking, a young person may want to live on the edge, feeling it a real adventure to join peers who are also experimenting with alcohol. With drinking, the young person feels more peer acceptance. Then, in the late teens and early twenties, more and more pressures are applied and the need for peer approval may never cease.

As Grace said, "Alcohol is the only mind–altering drug which one is asked to explain to peers why one is not using it."

8
Consequences of Alcohol Use in Colleges

The National Institute of Health (NIH) has done research, along with other investigators and the NIH reports that each year:

- ✓ 1,825 college students between ages 18 and 24 die from alcohol – related unintentional injuries, including motor-vehicle crashes. [30]
- ✓ 696,000 students between ages 18 and 24 are assaulted by another student who has been drinking. [31]
- ✓ 97,000 students between ages 18 and 24 report experiencing alcohol-related sexual assault or date rape. [31]
- ✓ Roughly 20% of college students meet the criteria for alcohol use disorder (alcoholism). [32]
- ✓ About 1 in 4 college students report academic consequences from drinking, including missing class, falling behind in class, doing poorly on exams or papers and receiving lower grades overall. [33]

As we consider the above numbers, how would we feel if interscholastic college football caused 1,825 deaths per year? We would discontinue college football.

But, with alcohol, we treat the problem differently. Some students and their parents want alcohol on campuses and colleges cater to students' wishes. If colleges do not cater to student's desires, colleges have fewer students, which means lower income to colleges. 1,825 alcohol deaths per year is a horrible number.

College administrators, alumnae, board and faculty members are struggling with how to take steps to decrease the tragic problems relating to student's alcohol use. Some colleges, such as Dartmouth, Brown, Swarthmore, University of Virginia, Stanford, Indiana and others have taken steps to combat the problem. [34]

One approach is to ban hard liquor on campuses, but any ban of any type of alcohol on campuses is very difficult to enforce. Since many students and their parents want to have alcohol available, college administrators are faced with a tough dilemma regarding how to control the use of this drug.

9
Betel Nuts

Someone once said that "all cultures need to have a drug." It is not easy to prove this, but, when one looks at the world, this may have a grain of truth.

Gaining more and more popularity now is the betel nut. [35] Seeds from the Areca Palm are treated and wrapped in leaves from the betel pepper plant, hence the name "betel nut." These are chewed and are very addictive.

These nuts are used in Thailand, Cambodia, India and other areas of southern Asia and the south Pacific, as well as in other areas of the world. Marketing is vigorous and officials who try to stop the use of betel nuts have difficult times — betel nuts make a lot of money. Marketers are now wrapping these items in bright colored wrappers to attract new segments of the population, especially children.

Does this remind us of marketing and flavoring of alcohol in the USA? Some producers of betel nuts add cloves, cinnamon, grated coconut, sugar and tobacco. These add to marketing efficiency.

Studies show that the use of betel nuts leads to mouth cancer, heart disease, diabetes, asthma and cirrhosis. [36]

Conclusion: Style and money dictate the use of many drugs.

Style and money. This can hold true for betel nuts and for alcohol. No question about it.

10
Boarding a Plane

Picture this: Let's say that you are boarding a plane. The cheerful flight attendant greets you, stating, "Have a great flight and remember that in the USA there are over 88,000 deaths each year due to commercial air crashes."

Well, you are smart. Of course, you know that there are NOT that number of yearly deaths due to airline crashes. Deaths due to airline crashes are very rare.

But, when we drink, we are taking part in an activity that kills over 88,000 people per year. Now let's assume that air crashes did indeed kill 88,000 people per year. That would be the same as 176 jumbo jets crashing yearly, killing all humans aboard. Horrible!

If that happened, would officials simply conduct seminars to encourage pilots to be more careful and to fly responsibly? No! Citizens would be aghast, and the air industry would likely ground jumbo jets, because to allow them to fly would be unthinkable.

But with the 88,000 alcohol deaths per year, we in the USA do not do much, except to provide gentle statements, at the end of alcohol ads, to drink responsibly. Also, some colleges give seminars and instructions to students on how to drink carefully and to not take risks with alcohol.

In the USA, we readily accept alcohol deaths, but we would never accept a similar number of air travel deaths. Never.

Why do we have different values regarding what types of deaths concern us?

11

What Does Alcohol Do?

Alcohol is classed as a depressant drug because it slows down the central nervous system with resultant behavior changes, psychological changes, muscular changes and altered thinking along with impaired judgment and impaired coordination.

It is distributed throughout the body, affecting almost every organ. It affects nearly every chemical process involving the brain and the nerve tissues in the brain. Alcohol is classified in medical textbooks as a drug, along with opioids, marijuana, cocaine, ecstasy, amphetamines and others.

Since our lives can be painful, alcohol can provide a temporary numbing of mental and emotional pain, as it depresses nerve tissues.

In very high doses, it can cause slowed breathing and death. [37]

Some alcohol users feel that it makes them less self–conscious in groups, with a "loosening of the tongue" so they can talk more freely. In the business world, this can be a disadvantage, in that at a business social function, the alcohol user may talk more than he/she should, giving away company secrets. In wartime, spies like to get "a few drinks into subjects" so that the subjects will have loose tongues and give away vital national information.

12

NFL, Breast Cancer and Alcohol

Breast cancer awareness is something that professional sports organizations in the USA frequently focus on. On certain days, players, coaches, officials and assistants wear articles that are pink to raise the public's awareness to breast cancer. Parts of the grass football fields have pink reminders to be aware of breast cancer. The National Football League (NFL) does this frequently. However, the NFL gives no money to breast cancer treatment or research.

Some say [38] that the NFL is interested, not so much in breast cancer, but in making women more sympathetic to the NFL, since far fewer than 50% of NFL television viewers are female. Also, since NFL players have been publicized for violence toward females, it is thought that the breast cancer awareness — pink display — might help women feel more sympathetic to the NFL in general. Perhaps the NFL is "throwing a rose" to women concerned about domestic violence.

This display of pink by the NFL has been called, by some news outlets, "The NFL's Pink Publicity Stunt." [38]

Here is an analysis: It is odd, indeed, that the NFL gives no money to breast cancer treatment or prevention. Breast cancer is a killer of 42,000 women per year. If the NFL wanted to focus on an American killer that is much more lethal than breast cancer, why would the NFL not focus on alcohol, which kills 88,000 Americans per year?

The answer is easy.

Social Alcohol

We can logically presume that the NFL will never focus on prevention of alcohol deaths because the NFL is made up of football club owners who gain huge revenues from alcohol sales at games.

It would appear that the more alcohol is sold and used at pro–games the happier the members of the NFL are and the more money they make. So, the NFL likely would not dare to even hint at cutting down on alcohol sales. It appears that they are more interested in making money than decreasing deaths.

In 2017 the NFL made a change in its rules which eliminated the prior ban of hard liquor ads on TV. For the first—time whiskey, vodka, rum and other spirits are allowed to advertise during NFL games. [6]

Of course, the NFL wants to increase revenue and the open door for liquor ads will, they assume, encourage more people to buy the product. If more people buy the product, will there be more resultant deaths and disability? Probably.

13
M and M Conferences

In many hospitals, there are periodic M and M (Mortality and Morbidity) Conferences where different patients' cases are reviewed.

These cases are taken apart, piece by piece and discussed at length by doctors. For example, if a patient has a surgery and there is a postoperative complication, this is defined as morbidity and this case is discussed in detail, to make decisions about how this morbidity could have been prevented.

Likewise, if a patient dies, this is defined as mortality and this case undergoes complex review. Hours are spent in these conferences, discussing mortality and morbidity. From these conferences we learn better ways to take care of patients.

We doctors just do not have M and M conferences when it comes to alcohol. We shrug our shoulders and we do not say much. When a patient or when a physician colleague has morbidity or even mortality from alcohol, we might say, "what a shame" as we walk away.

Interesting that we doctors spend so much time and agony on morbidity and mortality relating to patients' problems not relating to alcohol. If patients or doctors have alcohol related morbidity or mortality, we doctors barely give this subject the time of day.

14

The Lemming Effect

There are budding young executives who want to advance in their company. They feel that they had better be lemmings [39]* and use this drug called alcohol because if they do not use this drug like a lot of other budding young executives do and like their boss does, then they might be looked upon as being different. Then they might not advance as well in their company.

There are teenagers that see that other teens are using the drug alcohol, so they feel that they had better be lemmings and they had better use this drug so that they will be considered one of the group.

There are amateur softball players. The game is over. Seems like all of the players are going somewhere to use this drug. Well, if one player does not use this drug, that softball player might fear to be considered different and that would be not good. So, the softball player joins the other softball players, uses the drug and becomes a lemming. It is quite easy to be a lemming.

A construction worker is leaving the job at the end of the day. A bunch of nearby workers is heading to a place to get the drug. One worker does not want to be different. The lemming effect takes over.

* A modern urban legend says that lemmings perform mass suicides. As the Alaska Department of Fish and Game says, "Lemming Suicide Myth: Disney Film Faked Bogus Behavior." According to zoologist Gordon Jarrell, lemmings do join in mass movements. When they come to a body of water, they temporarily stop until they are so dense that they swim across. If they get wet to the skin they drown. [39]

The college freshman checks into the dorm. There is a nearby bunch of college freshmen preparing to go out and use this drug. The newly arrived freshman does not particularly want to use this drug, but he/she does not want to be different. So, it is quick for the student to become a lemming.

The above examples are prominent. A lot of us take part in the lemming effect with many of our actions. We simply want to be one of the crowd and we do not want to be labeled as standing alone. We want to do what others are doing.

This participation in the lemming effect is extremely important to us, no matter what our chronological age is and no matter how mature we are. We simply do not want to be different than others — we would rather be lemmings.

It does not take courage to be a lemming.

15
Personal Experience

The goal of this book is to draw very little on your personal experience or my personal experience with alcohol. Also, this book depends very little on your and my experience with friends, family and relatives relating to alcohol.

Why?

Because in this country of about 330 million people, your and my sample sizes are not significant. Our experiences with ourselves or with others are only anecdotes, only isolated events and to get conclusions, anecdotes do not carry weight. Anecdotes prove nothing.

All of us can relate stories of how different people or groups used alcohol. On first glance, these positive or negative accounts may seem impressive, but to draw reasonable conclusions, we need to study thousands and thousands of humans.

Very few Americans have the ability or the research money to do this. So, the numbers that are quoted in this book do not come from one person's observations, but from huge collections of data.

Example: It would be quite rare for one American citizen to do research to tell us the number of alcohol related deaths on college campuses. But the National Institute of Health (NIH) and Center for Disease Control (CDC) have complex methods to collect data and these are numbers that can help educate U S citizens.

So, someone may say, "My Uncle Charlie was such a horrible drunk that alcohol killed him." That statement is about one person and it means nothing, when we are making decisions.

Or, if a person says, "My Uncle Bill drank a lot, every day and it never bothered him. He is 88 years old and doing well." This statement, about one person, is not a valid one relating to decisions about alcohol.

Similarly, another statement could be: "My Uncle Joe never drank and as a result he never had any health problems and he never was involved with a drunk driving accident." Again, this statement about one person, means nothing.

To make decisions about alcohol, we need valid statistics about thousands of people. These statistics are available and are quoted in this book.

16
Outsourcing Our Behavior

It may be that we humans outsource our behavior more than we realize. I have done that a lot. Outsourcing our behavior to our environment is quite simple.

If all in a room are drinking and we enter the room and we drink, that may be outsourcing our behavior to our environment.

If all in a room are not drinking and we enter the room and do not drink, that could be outsourcing our behavior to our environment.

It is quite simple. We may do this more than we realize with activities other than alcohol. Alcohol can be a dangerous way to outsource our behavior.

The results can be quite unpleasant.

17
The P Word

As this book was being written, I have discussed its contents with others. Some have told me to remember that "prohibition simply did not work." (Yes, I just used the P word).

Of course, prohibition did not work. This book has nothing to do with prohibition. It did not work in the USA at all.

Somewhat interesting that in Russia, in 1914, Czar Nicholas instituted prohibition during the time of war. His goal was to try to keep the Russian soldiers sober during battle ... they were usually too drunk to fight, as they had been in previous wars. Prohibition failed in Russia, causing great problems, just as it did here in the USA.

This book encourages us to make accurate assessments of the drug alcohol, followed by personal, voluntary, individual decisions about the question: Is alcohol really a good drug, for me as a person and for society?

The P word will not be used again in this book.

Thank goodness!

18

Alcohol: The Drug That Changes Our Minds

David Dalke, a family counselor, said, "We can use any occasion as a reason to drink." [40]

 If we are happy with a raise in salary or a promotion, that is a reason. If we are discouraged after being fired, that is a reason. If we see an old friend after a long time of no contact, we can say, "let's go have a drink and catch up on things."

When my family and I lived in North Carolina, I attended a funeral of a peer who killed himself with an alcohol overdose. After the funeral, there was a social hour. The main beverage was alcohol ... as a matter of fact, non–alcoholic beverages were not served. Of the many people there, let's say that about 100 were consuming alcohol.

Simple arithmetic would say that for all of the adult males and females there who were drinking, between 8 and 9 guests would be alcoholics in the future. (As a matter of fact, with that many in the crowd, chances were good that some were already alcoholics.)

Interesting, when we recall that the reason for this social gathering was to honor a person who met his death by an alcohol overdose. We humans do interesting things.

19

If Only

Often, in conversations about alcohol morbidity and mortality (M and M) we often hear the statement ... "if only we Americans could ..." and several reasonable solutions are proposed. These "if only" proposals are fine, but it seems that often they are just left there and never carried out.

- ✓ If only it had not rained, we could have taken a trip.
- ✓ If only we could have avoided the bombing of Pearl Harbor, we would not have lost 30,000 lives.
- ✓ If only we had a better medication, we could prevent migraine headaches.
- ✓ If only he could have had more patience, he could have handled the challenges of life better.
- ✓ If only the intake of alcohol could be voluntarily decreased, the 88,000 alcohol related deaths per year would plummet and the 1825 college student alcohol related deaths per year would plummet.
- ✓ If only we could decrease alcohol consumption, the alcohol related child beatings and domestic beatings, plus certain alcohol related crimes would decrease greatly.
- ✓ If only we would take positive steps, we could get good results.

OK.

Social Alcohol

For this book and for this subject, let's avoid the *"if only"* phrase. It is off limits; because it can often be used as a helpless observation that the world would be fine *"if only."* So, for this book, instead of that *"if only"* phrase, let's use the words, *"let's do this."*

These three little words are not a lame, weak excuse to say let's just walk away from a very tough subject. When we examine the 88,000 unnecessary yearly deaths from alcohol, let's be positive and say, *"Let's do this."*

Or, another healthy phrase to say would be: "Here is a plan to approach the problem with vigor." Fine. We have agreed. *"If only"* will be used no more in these pages.

When the intake of alcohol is voluntarily decreased ...
- ✓ The 88,000 alcohol related deaths per year will plummet.
- ✓ The 1825 college student alcohol related deaths per year will plummet.
- ✓ The alcohol related child beatings and domestic beatings will decrease greatly.
- ✓ Certain alcohol related crimes will decrease greatly.

> *When we take positive steps,*
> *we will get good results.*

But, many of us have taken no action, so we sort of shrug our shoulders and accept the horrible 88,000 alcohol deaths per year. Some of us change the subject to a more pleasant one. We do not want to meddle with the status quo.

On the other hand, with desire, we *will* meddle with the status quo. To get results, it will take millions of lobbying dollars, millions of people voicing their concern and millions of citizens stating that they really did not need alcohol for an event, ballgame, or family gathering, or Christmas office party.

Millions of citizens will need to state that they did not need the crutch of alcohol to have a good time or a good day and these people will prove that their personalities were just fine and likely better without using a drug.

A distant parallel took place with tobacco, many decades ago. The dangers of tobacco related cancer were obvious, and many people stopped smoking, with a resultant healthier population. The rate of tobacco use in America is much less today, but still some people do smoke and the death rate from tobacco is significant.

In order to decrease smoking and its resultant blood vessel disease, heart disease, lung disease and lung cancer, the government has had several restrictions on tobacco advertising, which some states have followed. The government wisely has not made a law stating that tobacco could not be used, but its policies restricting certain tobacco ads have helped.

The door is open for the American public to help decrease the mortality and morbidity from alcohol, but the challenges are great. Alcohol manufacturers spend millions on lobbying and on advertising. Drunken behavior at athletic events is common, but if stadium concessions decreased or stopped alcohol sales, the alcohol distributors would raise great objections. The obstacles to progress are great but obstacles can be confronted and surmounted.

Social Alcohol

During World War II, 405,000 American deaths occurred, or roughly 100,000 deaths per year. Compare that death rate to the yearly death rate in the USA from alcohol ... 88,000 deaths per year. Some authors state the alcohol death rate is 100,000 per year [3].

Compare these yearly deaths from alcohol, to yearly death rates from war. We fought bravely, and we sacrificed in WW II. We lost 100,000 humans per year for a great cause ... to have a free country. Now we are losing almost the same number of people per year from alcohol, but unlike WW II, the alcohol deaths per year are not limited ... which was the case in WW II ...in 1945, the war deaths just stopped.

It is a tragedy that the alcohol deaths are about the same per year as the war, but the alcohol deaths just keep continuing, year after year, far beyond the "limit" of WW II deaths.

The war deaths we accepted so we could remain free. The alcohol deaths we accept because these deaths are due to a recreational drug ... alcohol. What kind of logic is this? Does this really make any sense?

There are some definite, positive steps to take, which can get results. Check out the chapters in the Subject Index under "Next Steps" for some ideas.

20

Could a Decrease in Alcohol Use Help Society?

Of course, it would help society. That is a slam dunk. Let's say that we had a "Day of No Alcohol Use in the USA." You know, sort of like "Bike–to–Work Day." Ridiculous? No. Possible? Yes.

If we had one day of no alcohol use, there would automatically be no alcohol related car crashes and resultant deaths that day. About 28 lives would be saved, immediately. Is 28 a trivial number? No. Especially if you or a loved one is one of the 28.

Think about that number. What would we do, in this country, if we had 28 deaths per day from golf, or city league basketball, or bowling? The answer is a no brainer. We would, without a doubt, discontinue golf, or city league basketball, or bowling. Now, here is the catch — if we did decide to decrease recreational alcohol usage, there could be multitudes of objections from industry and from other sources.

21
Disease and Deaths

In the USA, if we had an illness such as measles, strep infection, or meningitis, that caused 88,000 deaths per year, our country would be up in arms. We would be doing everything possible to prevent this disease.

Alcohol kills 88,000 people per year. What are we doing about it?

Actually, we are just selling more alcohol. Granted, we have a few signboards stating, "Don't Drink and Drive" or at the end of an alcohol TV ad, there could be the statement "Drink responsibly."

But, overshadowing these admonitions, we are advertising alcohol greatly in the print media, on television and on the radio. Our goal, as a country, seems to be: Sell more alcohol. It appears that the death rate does not matter ...we just want to keep alcohol sales up.

22

Dangerous Deception

Hiding the Evidence of Adverse Drug Effects

An article in the New England Journal of Medicine by J. Avorn [41] had the above title. The first sentence stated, "Recently there was a day of infamy for Merck Drug Company."

On a recent date, Merck announced that they were withdrawing from the market a drug (Vioxx) which had been used for five years in over 20 million patients. The reason for the withdrawal was that this drug doubled the risk of heart attack and stroke.

Merck steadfastly denied that Vioxx increased the risk of heart attack while the drug was on the market, making a huge profit for Merck. While denying the adverse and dangerous effects of Vioxx, Merck financed a study, done by Avorn, to check on possible increased dangers of Vioxx.

When Avorn reported the dangerous findings to Merck, Merck denied the findings. This appeared to be an obvious coverup. Finally, Merck took the drug off of the market, because of much pressure from authorities. The public had been deceived long enough.

With a different drug, Avorn reported that in September 1982, six Chicago people died after taking acetaminophen (Tylenol) that had been laced with cyanide. This horrible tragedy riveted the country's attention for months.

Social Alcohol

Avorn writes that we should be able to muster at least a fraction of that acetaminophen concern to address the horrible problems relating to drugs, promoted by drug companies, that can sicken or kill thousands of patients.

Of all of the drugs in the USA, alcohol is a second only to tobacco with its death rate. Somehow, we citizens were horrified about the six Tylenol deaths, but those six deaths paled in comparison to the 88,000 alcohol deaths per year, including the 1825 yearly alcohol deaths on college campuses. [31]

We Americans focus our attention on unique subjects. With guidance from the press, we seem to focus our concerns on the "tragedy of the day," which at one time was 6 Tylenol deaths.

The alcohol industry likely will not quote to us yearly alcohol deaths, while emphasizing in their ads the pleasure resulting from alcohol. Alcohol companies are participating in dangerous deception with their expensive promotions of their dangerous drug.

23

Deaths from Illnesses

Cervical cancer causes 6,000 deaths per year in the USA. In 2014, breast cancer caused 41,211 deaths. [1]

We vigorously screen for and we make every effort to prevent cervical cancer by doing pap smears. Similarly, we make every effort to prevent breast cancer, using mammograms and other methods. These cancers, added together, cause far fewer deaths than the deaths due to alcohol, which total 88,000 per year.

We spend huge amounts of money to prevent cervical cancer and breast cancer. How much money is spent in preventing alcohol problems? Very little. But, we keep advertising alcohol. We keep promoting it, pushing it and glorifying it.

Why do we do this? Other than money, other than style and other than peer pressure, why do we keep pushing and promoting alcohol?

24
Theology and Alcohol

There is no attempt whatsoever in this book to analyze alcohol and its relation to the many theologies of the world. That writing would involve many volumes and this brief book does not attempt that.

Instead, this book touches on only one common statement that is heard in the United States relating alcohol to theology. That statement, often heard, is, "Jesus drank wine, so it drinking alcohol is OK."

A reply to that concept is:

It may be that wine was used in the day of Jesus because the water was polluted and unfit to drink, causing sickness. If we are going to use Jesus as our standard and yardstick for our actions, let's not cherry pick his actions, using one action of Jesus as justification on what we already like to do. If we use Jesus as our yardstick, let's be fair and copy him in all of his activities. This could be unpleasant indeed.

We would sleep on mats, would never use air conditioning, we would wear sandals and a robe, eat fish cooked on an open fire, only eat foods used in that day.

We would not get immunizations. If sick, we would take no medications. We would not have dental care. We would avoid marriage because Jesus was single. We would walk everywhere, not using cars. We would stop on our walks, to give talks to crowds about theology.

If we had a gall bladder attack or an attack of appendicitis, we would not have surgery and we might die. If we had a broken leg, we would have no medical care and we might become lame for the rest of our lives.

No ...it is not logical to use Jesus as our yardstick for alcohol use. If we use Jesus as our yardstick, let's be fair and make it all or nothing.

Phil Rogers [42] recently wrote a paper on the use of alcohol in organized churches. Rogers referred to Jewett, who in his book "The Two Wine Theory" [43], stated that Biblical references to wine included two types of wine — one, called yayin, which contained alcohol and the other called tirosh, containing no alcohol.

Rogers made the point that at the Passover meal [44] there is mention of unleavened bread and wine. Rogers assumed that this wine was tirosh, with no alcohol. Fermented wine would have required a leavening agent so, Rogers assumes, in referring to Jewett's book, that the wine at that meal was grape juice.

S. Hamilton mentions in his publication [45] that some liquids in the Bible referred to as wine were non—alcoholic. Hamilton explains yayin and tirosh are from Hebrew; oinos and gleukos are from Greek; and vioum is from Latin.

Tirosh and gleukos are always non—fermented grape juice but they are translated in most Bibles as wine. The other three words, yayin, oinos and vioum, could either be fermented or non—fermented grape juice. We simply do not know.

25

Criticism is of the Drug, Not the People

Some who read these pages might say, "Why criticize the person who drinks alcohol?"

That is absolutely NOT what these pages are doing. This book is not putting down humans who drink.

The concern is about the drug and what harm it can do. This point must be emphasized repeatedly. The people who drink are good people and nice people. These good people and nice people, when drinking, can encounter big problems.

That is what can happen with this dangerous drug.

26
Words from Annie Grace

Annie Grace, a recovering alcoholic, wrote a book titled "This Naked Mind." [29] Here are some quotes from her book:

About social alcohol: Annie says: "Alcohol is the only drug on earth that one needs to justify not using. Today's society has conditioned your mind to believe alcohol provides pleasure, enjoyment and support — that it is vital to social situations and stressful situations alike."

In her book, Annie reverses that false belief about alcohol. Annie mentions other false beliefs that society may embrace, one of which is:

"Alcohol provides enjoyment, relief and is the key to social situations — a party really can't be a party without booze — it makes us funnier and more attractive, while it relieves stress and boredom."

Annie shows that this is false. She states, "Everyone who drinks ... can be on the path to alcohol dependence ... over time, with the right level of exposure, anyone can develop a physical dependence on alcohol. This message is not popular; it flies in the face of our thriving alcohol industry, our social dependence on the drug and the attitudes of 'regular' and 'responsible' drinkers."

Regarding children, Annie says, "We are unintentionally conditioning our children. We are programing them to believe that their lives will not be complete without drinks in their hands."

Social Alcohol

About acquired tastes, Mrs. Grace says, "'You just have to acquire the taste' is the great deceit that lures new drinkers in."

Annie Grace tells of a friend who is French, "Her parents encouraged her to have sips of wine at dinner from the age of eight. She never liked it and would tell them so, but they would insist on at least one sip, telling their daughter to just wait and see — she would like it when she is older." Sure enough, she is now older and now she drinks a lot every night.

When we take our first sips and almost gag, there's often someone there to reassure us, "Alcohol is an acquired taste and we should not give up. We will grow to like it."

27

Incidence of Alcoholism

In the USA, the incidence of alcoholism among all adult males over age 18 is 12.4%, while the incidence among all adult females is 4.9%. Considering all sexes, the incidence of alcoholism among adults is 8.5% [8].

If a person does not drink, that person will not be an alcoholic. For persons who do not drink, the incidence of alcoholism is zero. If a person drinks, the 12.4% chance of alcoholism for males and the 4.9% chance of this problem for females represent great risks. This means that alcohol usage has potential future problems that are grave.

To compare — if one uses frequent air travel, how would one feel if one were told that there would always be a 12% chance for a severe, possibly fatal disease for men, and an 4.9% chance of severe, possibly fatal disease for women, due to air travel?

How casually would we take air travel, if this were the case? But it appears that many humans look at alcohol use just as casually as air travel, ignoring the future risks of alcohol use. Another way to look at alcohol usage is: Of all men who drink, there is a one in 8 chance that they will become alcoholics. Of all women who drink, there is a one in 20 chance that they will become alcoholics. Those are frightful numbers for a drug that is just for recreation and not necessary for any other use.

28
Sports Events and Alcohol

Journalists from the Associated Press and *USA Today* reported [46] that alcohol, primarily beer, is vigorously marketed at American ballparks, despite rowdy and even criminal behavior that may result. The reports stated that beer and baseball are tightly bound.

Researchers did breathalyzer tests on 362 fans, leaving 13 baseball games and three NFL games and found that 8% of the departing fans were legally drunk. That 8%, when multiplied by the thousands of fans attending games nationwide, leads to a staggering number.

Reporters and researchers asked eight professional teams for arrest for drunkenness statistics at their ballparks and none of the teams provided answers. The researchers concluded that alcohol at sports events definitely leads to problems and despite this, alcohol is vigorously promoted and sold at sporting events.

One reason for this is that alcohol companies can be key sponsors of stadiums and their teams. Stadiums get sponsorship and money from the alcohol companies and, when they get the money from alcohol industries, they serve and advertise the products and of course there are large revenues from alcohol sales at each sports complex.

If 8% is a marker, then athletic facilities apparently are not concerned about that 8% number of drunken spectators. If fifty thousand are at a sporting event, this could mean that four thousand spectators are drunk. That is an impressive number.

29
Reaction Time

The Mayo Clinic reported [47] that any amount of alcohol can impair reaction time. For example, one beer may not elevate the blood alcohol concentration (BAC) a lot. But even though the BAC is below the legal limit, reaction time can still be impaired and driving a car could be dangerous to you and others on the road.

This may be part of the reason why, in England, Dr. Sally Davies, the Chief Medical Officer of that country, stated that as a national policy, there is no safe amount of alcohol to consume. [9] This statement from England does not agree with the often–heard statement, "A little alcohol is OK, as long as I am not drunk and as long as I do not harm someone."

Since I am a sports fan, I have often wondered about this while watching pro games. I have not ever seen alcohol in a baseball dugout or on the football sidelines or on the bench in a basketball game.

It would be a monumental task to interview a hundred or so sports teams to ask them why we do not see alcohol for players to use during the game. Without such a complex research project, my assumption is that the coaches and owners do not want to impair reaction time, thinking skills and physical dexterity of their players as they make crucial athletic decisions. Of course, there are, on the sidelines, non–alcoholic sports drinks and water for the athletes.

Social Alcohol

If there are readers who feel that my assessments about no alcohol consumed during games by pro players are not correct, help me learn by contacting me by email. My email address is on my website listed on the outside of the back cover.

I have a good friend who likes a couple of beers now and then. At the end of the evening, he asks his wife to drive him and their small children home. He feels that this is fine as he is not driving, hence no car accident. The problem with this thinking is that if there is a car crash and his wife is seriously injured, or if one of his children has a medical emergency like a seizure, not related to a potential car crash, his reaction time, thinking skills and dexterity are hampered, making him less efficient in any type of emergency.

30
Christmas Party

Ike: Jake, I just don't see the point of this. This social scene is weird. Our workplace is a fairly reasonable place. We get along all right and we do work that is quite excellent. Our work ethic is tremendous, and we have no personality problems, which is amazing.

But then our annual Christmas party came around. I just don't get it. At our Christmas party there was a bunch of alcohol flowing. People acted weird and did dumb and stupid things.

Some people insulted others. Some people got skunk–drunk and a few people just got pretty well greased.

Well, I just don't understand this. We are a reasonable bunch of people, so we have a party and we have to use a drug to have fun?

Jake: Well, this is sort–of a custom, Ike. At Christmas parties, like, it is sort–of accepted that you have some booze as part of the celebration.

Ike: As part of a celebration? We have to have a drug to celebrate? Can't you celebrate without a drug?

Jake: Well, it's just sort–of the way it is in this country.

Ike: Hmm. Seems weird to me.

Jake: Yep, it is weird, but that's just the way it is.

Social Alcohol

Ike: Next year, I'm going to host a Christmas party. It's going to be alcohol–free and drug–free.

Jake: Someone might tell you that is different than the established norm.

Ike: Fine. I want us to depend on the human personality rather than upon other stuff. We'll depend on our human personalities to have fun.

Jake: Good idea.

31

We Americans Do Interesting Things

18% of Americans believe that the sun rotates around the earth. Well, this is interesting, because if this misconception continues, it goes right along with other interesting things that Americans believe.

For example, the number of Americans who die each year from tobacco use is 480,000, but some Americans continue tobacco use, feeling that it is really OK, ignoring the death rate.

Similarly, many Americans ignore the 88,000 alcohol deaths per year, continuing to use the stylish approach, thinking that alcohol is really a good drug.

We Americans do interesting things.

32

Humans Do Odd Things

We have anti–drug programs. We have drug rehab centers. Signs near schools say, "Drug Free Zone." Bumper stickers say, "Just Say No." Many organizations say, "Dare to Say No" to drugs.

This is all well and good. But why do we not say, "No to all drugs?" We advocate saying "no" to cocaine, "no" to tobacco and "no" to speed. We accept these as agents to which we should say, "no." Well, why not say, "no" to alcohol also?

Society has put the drug alcohol in a different category. We teach college students to use alcohol in moderation and to have a designated driver and to use the drug alcohol very carefully. We remind citizens that if they drink not to drive.

Isn't it odd we do not use these concepts relating to alcohol to other drugs. We never say, "If you use cocaine, use it sparingly" and we do not say, "If you use speed, remember to get a designated driver." We do not say that if tobacco is used, "Just be very careful, it could be dangerous."

Our society can be so hypocritical. We teach people to use alcohol "sparingly and responsibly and in an adult way." At the same time, we teach people to not use cocaine, speed, tobacco and other drugs at all. All of us really ought to get on the same page.

We are weird in what we teach. If we educate and if we advertise to use alcohol carefully, which kills 88,000 humans per year in the USA, then why do we instruct the avoidance of cocaine, which kills only 5,000 per year? Similarly, why do we teach and encourage and advertise alcohol use, when we teach avoidance of heroin, which kills only 13,000 per year?

We humans do odd things, indeed.

33
The Economics of Alcohol

Parts of America love alcohol. Many in America love the economics of alcohol. Some Americans love the tax revenue from alcohol and many retailers love alcohol sales. America and alcohol may be "just where they want to be." America and alcohol are very comfortable bedfellows when money is so important.

When it comes to economics and money making, many people profit from alcohol in an ironic, sad way. Since a lot of Americans profit from alcohol sales, a lot of people do not want to meddle with this very happy "good deal" that makes some citizens financially happy.

Can you picture the scene in a boardroom of a nationwide alcohol beverage company if the C E O announced that he/she was very concerned about the yearly American deaths due to alcohol and if he/she suggested that this company should promote a decrease in sales so that less alcohol would be consumed in the USA?

What would the members in the boardroom say? What would the stockholders say?

The responses are pretty predictable.

34
Fact Based Actions

In medicine, there is a concept called "evidence– based medicine." That means that we do not do anything in medicine unless we have evidence that what we are doing is correct, backed up by scientific data.

For example, many decades ago, tonsillectomies were done quite often as routine operations on children with no symptoms because it was thought that the operations were a "good idea." Now, science has shown that every child does not need a tonsillectomy. In fact, the operation can carry with it major complications.

The same reasoning holds true for alcohol. For decades, we consumers thought, "Well, alcohol does no harm." That is incorrect. Indeed, alcohol often causes harm and there could be a possible analogy between routine tonsillectomy because "everyone is doing it" and alcohol consumption because "everyone is doing it."

35

Revolvers, Society and Alcohol

Let's face it. society and humanity — that is, people in general — have not progressed to the point that we can place a loaded revolver on the kitchen table and leave it there all of the time. We just cannot do that; it is not wise. Think of what might happen if a person happened to be having a terrible day, walked by the revolver and had a sudden terrible impulse to do harm.

Similarly, society has proven that it cannot handle the concept of making social and recreational alcohol part of our everyday life. The death rate (88,000 deaths per year) is just too high and the tragedy rate (bad things short of death) is also too high. The latter include paralyzed humans after car wrecks, loss of limbs, child abuse, rapes, beatings and severe domestic abuse, plus other examples of morbidity.

We generally do not keep loaded revolvers on kitchen tables, in most families. But often, families have alcohol at their fingertips — in the refrigerator or real close by.

36
Parents Teaching Children to Drink

Often, intelligent, responsible, parents state, "I will teach my children early, at a young age, to drink carefully and responsibly, so that they will not be problem drinkers later in life."

This logic is a myth. The World Health Organization [48] quotes published studies that prove this idea wrong. More than one study has shown that early initiation of alcohol use, before age 14, is associated with increased risks for alcohol dependence and use later in life.

37

Some Populations Cannot Handle Alcohol

We know that sometimes, one person can go throughout life having a small amount of daily alcohol and alcohol does not kill that person — that person dies from something else. But we must remember, that person is advertising to many other people that alcohol is a good drug. Unfortunately, the vulnerable people who are influenced by that person's advertising of alcohol might not be so fortunate.

When we examine some large populations, like the USA, England or Russia, it is obvious that some large populations simply cannot handle the drug alcohol. The abuse rates and the mortality and morbidly rates are terrible. The death rate of 88,000 per year is a reminder that many in our culture in the USA cannot handle alcohol.

Therefore, we could consider a "gradual phasing out" of alcohol beverages. This will take time and it cannot be done by legislation (remember the horrible events of Prohibition in the USA). This phasing out can be done quietly, as persons simply stop using the drug.

When we realized that stagecoaches were no longer needed, we gradually phased them out. When we realize that we do not need alcohol, we can phase it out.

We can do with the drug alcohol what we did with tobacco. In the thirties and forties, tobacco was highly accepted. When we considered the unfortunate results of tobacco use, we gradually began to phase it out. Today, tobacco has been eliminated from many parts of our culture.

We could most certainly do that with alcohol. It could be, actually, quite simple.

38

Pick A Number

Let's play a game, a simple one. Let's pick a number — 88,000 — the most often quoted number representing deaths in the USA each year from alcohol. Some authorities [3] say that the number is over 100,000 deaths per year, but we will use 88,000, the most often quoted figure.

Year by year, we know that the 88,000 number does not change much. Our concern about that number can be a doctor giving a wink and a nod to a patient, carefully reminding the patient that alcohol has some disadvantages. Or, another American approach is to present multimillion dollar TV displays advertising alcohol, with quiet careful admonitions at the ends of the ads to drink responsibly.

Now, what would be the reaction of the citizens of the USA, if professional football activity resulted in 88,000 deaths per year? Would we say, in a quiet way to the players, to play responsibly? No, we might discontinue the sport of football.

Or, consider NASCAR. If these car races caused 88,000 deaths per year, would we issue a wink and a nod, as we do with alcohol, reminding the drivers, that there could be some disadvantages and they might want to cut down on their speed? No ... NASCAR might be eliminated.

And, we must remember the jumbo jet story. To repeat, that would be the situation if 176 jumbo jets in this country crashed in a year, killing all passengers on the planes (88,000 deaths). Would we send a quiet memo to airlines, humbly asking the airlines to be very careful and to fly responsibly? No ...of course not. We would likely eliminate jumbo jet travel, using different types of airplanes.

We in the USA pick what we want to be concerned about and we pick which numbers we ignore. We often ignore the 88,000 alcohol deaths each year. Why? Alcohol is a huge money–making industry, which provides financial gain to many, many Americans.

We Americans have chosen to leave the alcohol deaths just as they are. We have chosen not to meddle with that death rate — meddling could be very unpopular because of massive profits coming to the alcohol industry.

The alcohol yearly death rate is pretty constant, and the death rate keeps ticking away, year by year, like a dependable clock. Yearly alcohol deaths are a tragedy and they do not stop. In the USA, by doing nothing, we are encouraging these deaths by looking the other way.

It is not a bit convenient or popular for us to address the yearly tragic alcohol deaths.

39

Oh Boy! Here's How to Be Manly!

This book's goal is to concentrate on reason and logic in a clear, dignified way. But what the heck! Let's introduce a little sarcasm, just for fun.

OK. Here are excerpts of the exact wording circulated by a large, mainline, well respected church: (Name has been changed.)

Email title line: "Say a MANLY goodbye to Pastor Joe Smith!"

Body of email: "As Pastor Joe moves away ...we need to say goodbye to Joe in the proper way – with beer and food."

OK. Email quote is over. Let's now consider the email, sent from this church. The hidden message could be and yes, I have added some sarcasm:

Hey men ... if you want to be true men, come and join us for a few beers. And men, if you have early teenage sons who see this message and if they want to join us, do remind them that they are just not old enough to do this manly thing. In a few years, they can start drinking beer legally, like the rest of us, then they can really qualify as men.

And dads, when you tell your sons these things, remember that your words are sure fire ways to propel your sons into some serious drinking. Remind your sons several times that drinking is the manly thing to do ... the church said so ... in their email.

Oh yes, dads, remember to tell your sons that when they embark on this manly endeavor, whether they are underage or not, there is a good chance that they will become alcoholics ... one in eight men who drink do become alcoholics.

But, no problem. Just tell your sons that there is always Alcoholics Anonymous (AA). And Dads, remember to tell your sons that one–month residential programs are horribly expensive.

OK. Author's sarcasm is over ... but the serious points have been made.

Mothers and daughters, this chapter applies equally to you. Please take it to heart!

40
New Trend

A new trend could occur — a trend that it is cool not to drink. This trend should NOT be carried out with any suggestion or a hint of arrogance or superiority. It should proceed with a measure of newness, fun and adventure. If large numbers of people do this, we would decrease the yearly alcohol related deaths.

41
It's Deceptively Simple

It is really quite simple, it is deceptively simple, to decrease and even eliminate the deaths and pain that result from social alcohol. It is so simple, it is hard to believe.

The plan is this: We simply stop using social alcohol. Can we do it overnight? Likely not. Humanity does not snap its fingers and change its behavior overnight. It took society some time to stop the habit of dueling and we did not gain women's suffrage quickly. And slavery in this country did not rapidly disappear.

But with alcohol, the goal can easily be achieved. Society can begin to decrease its consumption of alcohol and over a reasonable period of time, we can stop its consumption. Many communities, businesses and individuals have done this with tobacco. When presented with this concept, some might say, "Oh, it is impossible. It is just not practical. Besides, a little social alcohol is certainly okay."

The answer to that objection is quite straightforward. The answer is: "What is the point of using social alcohol anyway?" Is it to make a human feel more relaxed? Is the point to make conversation easier to come by in social groups? Is the point to satisfy an addiction?

If these are the reasons to use alcohol, none of them are legitimate. These reasons do not make sense. Consider alcohol related traffic deaths: If we, as a society, stopped consuming alcohol for 24 hours, we, for the adjacent 24 hours, would have no alcohol related traffic fatalities; we would have eliminated many useless deaths.

42
Just One Beer

Some people honestly say, "Just one beer is all that I ever have. I like this, and it really doesn't matter, because one beer will never do any harm."

This statement is interesting. Some individuals can go through their lives, having just one beer per day or per week. They do not become alcoholics and they do not have an incident such as a car wreck or a terrible event. However, this person, if a male, has a 12.4% chance of becoming an alcoholic. That 12.4% is a staggering number and it is a massive risk to take.

If they had never had that periodic one beer, they would not have had that one out of eight chances of becoming an alcoholic. Also, that "one beer person" is a continuous advertisement to all that alcohol is a good and desirable thing. Young people, peers and vulnerable individuals could use the one beer person as an example and get started using alcohol. And each male who begins this drug has the 12.4% chance of becoming an alcoholic.

One out of 8! 12.4% is a rough and undesirable number. So, the phrase "just one beer" is not as harmless as it sounds. The "one beer person" may not be able to handle it and the one beer later becomes four beers and that person may become an alcoholic, harming others with the drug. Also, the one beer person should remember that one beer can definitely affect behavior, thinking and physical dexterity. During an emergency, these changes can be crucial.

Maybe that is why, as we observe pro athletes and doctors in the operating room, we do not see them having "just one beer" at break time, during time outs or between surgical cases.

I have been involved with surgeries lasting 12 or more hours and never have I seen a doctor "stop for a beer." In the doctors' dressing room, in preparation for an upcoming surgery or after a surgery is finished, there is no alcohol. There is a good reason for that.

In a courtroom, the case may last several hours. Do we see the judge or the lawyers or the jury sipping "just one beer" during the proceedings? No! They want to be as sharp as possible and they understand that one beer could alter their thinking and reasoning skills.

43

Influenza Deaths and Alcohol Deaths

Influenza causes many deaths each year in the United States. The Center for Disease Control (CDC) acknowledges the difficulty in knowing the exact number of deaths per year. However, in 2016 the CDC estimated that there were between 12,000 and 56,000 deaths from influenza in 2015. [49]

We correctly advise people to obtain their flu shots which prevent many deaths.

In the same year, there were 88,000 deaths from alcohol. Yet, we continue to vigorously advertise and promote the use of more and more alcohol.

Is our logic flawed?

44

Really Not a Dangerous Substance?

Alcohol really is not a dangerous substance? Just go to the ballgame and have 1 or 2 beers. This never hurts anybody? Well, why does the management of the ballpark agree to stop selling alcohol after the 7th inning? Could it be because this really is not a harmless substance?

If the ballpark owners continued to sell alcohol through the entire game, they would certainly have more sales. So why do they stop the sales after the seventh inning?

Likely, the reason could be very simple. Even one drink, i.e., one beer, can cause a blood alcohol level that can impair judgment, mental quickness and physical skills in some people.

So, it is a wise idea for the ballpark to stop selling alcohol after the 7th inning. They have a good reason for this — alcohol is not simply a harmless substance.

45

Tough Results

In 2015 there were 10,265 deaths in the USA due to alcohol impaired car crashes. These accounted for almost a third of all of the traffic deaths in the USA. [12]

All of these deaths were easily preventable. This means that 28 deaths per day, due to alcohol related car crashes, are preventable. This is the same as 20 jumbo jets crashing in one year, with all the passengers dying.

What would our society do if we had 20 jumbo jets crashing in one year, with all of the passengers dying? Our society might scream bloody murder and all jumbo jets might be grounded.

But with the alcohol related car crashes, we as a society barely consider the problem. We do not even consider it enough to shrug our shoulders. Often, we simply are not interested.

66% of marital abuse and violence is due to alcohol [50] while some report that 96% of assailants used alcohol at the time of the attack. [51]

All of the above are tough, tough results.
Very tough.
And very sad.

46
Town of 100,000

Question: If you approached a town of 100,000 in the United States and this town had never heard of beverage alcohol or social alcohol, would you want to introduce it to this town?

Would it do that town good? Would it help the quality of life in the town? Remember, of all the men and women in this town who begin social alcohol, 4.9% of women will become alcoholics and 12.4% of men will do the same. Of all of the social drinkers, 50% will have alcohol related incidents, such as car wrecks, domestic abuse and other trauma.

So, will it be good to introduce alcohol to this town?

47

Fashion Determines Substance Use

Substance use, like carpets and hats, obeys the laws of fashion. (Author unknown) Society seems to accept this statement much of the time.

For example, several decades ago, ladies in the USA dipped snuff — not so fashionable today. Several decades ago, American baseball players commonly chewed tobacco — not done today. General MacArthur in WW II was known for his famous corncob pipe — we do not see military officers smoking pipes today.

Today in Asia, the betel nut, quite addictive, is placed in the mouth — and can be a gift of goodwill at weddings and prominent social functions. The betel nut is sold commonly on the street and many people use it daily.

In Africa, leaves of the plant khat are placed in the mouth — khat is addictive, used by many males for many hours per day.

In the average American social group, one does not see prominent use of khat or the betel nut. These substances are not really fashionable here. One can speculate how it would be if the host of a highly regarded dinner and social function, say a fund raiser for a large city charity, would change the custom.

Instead of serving many choices of alcohol, considered fashionable, how would it be if a khat leaf was at the place setting of every dinner guest, along with a betel nut? These would replace the expected wine glasses.

Likely, the unsuspecting dinner guests would not only be surprised or taken aback and some would be offended. The betel nuts and khat leaves would be defined as not fashionable, unlike the expected alcohol.

Yes, fashion does determine the substances that we use. It is a bigtime determinant.

Actually, khat is illegal in the United States. Khat contains two central nervous system stimulants: cathinone — a Schedule I drug under the Federal Controlled Substances Act — and cathine — a Schedule IV drug. Cathinone is the principal active stimulant; its levels are highest in fresh khat. [52]

48

Tolstoy

Leo Tolstoy, the famous Russian author, wrote an essay with the title "Why Do Men Stupefy Themselves?" This actually is not one of his best works. It is rife with opinion, anecdotes and rather impulsive statements. His conclusion is that alcohol indeed is a destructive agent for humanity.

Tolstoy also makes the point (a good one), that we need to ask the question "why do we men (and women) stupefy ourselves?"

The answer may be that a lot of our peers are doing it. If our peers were not stupefying themselves, we probably would not either. Why do we humans need something to change our thinking and to make us unable to think clearly? Why do we seek a substance to provide us with a different state of mind?

Interesting — betel nuts, tobacco, alcohol, khat, marijuana. All of these things can and do stupefy us and they can change the way that we feel about life. In different world cultures, different stupefying agents seem to be characteristic.

In our culture, alcohol is a favorite stupefying agent.

49
Vioxx and Alcohol

As mentioned in Chapter 22, "Dangerous Deception," in 2005, the Federal Government took a drug off the market because of its dangers.

A new drug, Vioxx, was introduced by a drug company. Its use was to relieve pain. This new drug worked pretty well for pain relief. But it was shown that, over a five–year period, Vioxx increased deaths from heart attacks, ranging from 5,000 deaths per year to 11,000 deaths per year. These deaths were tragic, not necessary and Vioxx was correctly removed from use in the USA. [53]

Now ... let's compare Vioxx, causing 5,000 to 11,000 deaths per year, to alcohol, causing at least 88,000 deaths per year. Vioxx did have a solid medical indication to relieve severe pain from arthritis.

Alcohol, on the other hand, is a recreational drug, just like marijuana or tobacco and its reason for use is recreation. It has no medical indication for its use like Vioxx did.

Alcohol causes many more deaths per year than Vioxx and Vioxx was taken off the market because of its dangers. Our American society agreed that Vioxx was removed because of its dangers. We Americans are doing basically nothing about the dangers of the recreational drug alcohol.

Our thinking is interesting, to say the least.

50
Victimized?

Once a person told me that their family member was victimized by a disease. The disease that afflicted the family member, they explained, was alcoholism and their family had a genetic trait that contributed to family members becoming alcoholics.

There are several ways to look at this. If that human had not chosen to be a drinker to begin with, then that human would never have been victimized by this "disease." The disease of alcoholism is a result of a definite choice. A human chooses to drink, a human drinks too much, a human is an alcoholic. That is simple.

Victimized by a disease? We must be careful with that phrase. Any human who chooses to drink has a significant chance of becoming an alcoholic. That is a no brainer. Now, this is in no way pointing the finger of judgment at a person who is an alcoholic; this is not making any type of accusation directed to an alcoholic. It is simply recognizing a fact, which is: If a person does not drink, that person will never be an alcoholic. That fact is very plain.

Is there a genetic tendency to be more prone to succumb to alcoholism? Yes. [54] Scientists are studying this. But the bottom line is that if a person does have a genetic tendency to become an alcoholic, if that person chooses to not drink, that person will not be an alcoholic.

It is a choice.

A simple choice.

51
Who Has It Helped?

One scholar who studied alcohol and its positive and negative effects asked the following question: "Look around you and look at your life. Look at your acquaintances. Look at your friends, family and peers. Name the people you know or acquainted with who have shown that alcohol has had definite positive benefits on their lives."

When one attempts to do this, one can see a lot of individuals who have shown very negative influences from alcohol. When one looks for people who have received positive benefits from alcohol, these people are hard to find.

One might argue that alcohol merchants or those who are full time in the alcohol industry have profited financially from alcohol. This is a hard argument to defend since alcohol is a potent drug. One could just as easily state that tobacco, marijuana, or cocaine merchants could get positive results from their sales of those drugs.

So, the argument that those employed in the alcohol industry gain positive benefits really does not hold. Since the United States and Great Britain, as well as the World Health Organization (See "Advice and Opinions," page 12), have removed their earlier policy statements that small amounts of alcohol could have possible benefits to the heart, this old advice is no longer valid and is not a reason to drink.

52

The Seductive Siren with a Smile

Alcohol, of course, is a drug. That is a fact and it has never been questioned. Standard medical textbooks classify it as a drug. It is always listed in the drug section along with cocaine, heroin and other drugs. [3] [55]

However, our culture has decided that it will be known as a "drug with a smile."

This idea of a "drug with a smile" has been fueled by advertisements. That is, this drug has a "come hither" approach to both men and to women. It smiles at males, females, teens and adults. It has a siren–like quality which causes people to respond to it as if they owe it to themselves to use this exciting liquid. This is sad, but true.

Friends and alcohol ads say, in essence, "get on board and experience this pleasure, like the rest of us. Do not deprive yourself of this great feeling."

This is too bad, but it is true. The fact is, this drug can have dangerous results and extremely uncomfortable end points. Sad — and very true.

53
Taking Chances

When we think of "taking chances," most 25 to 35–year old young men would likely not consider it wise to perform any activity, for business or pleasure, that had a 12.4% chance of resulting in extreme lifelong illness or even death. These are somber odds. However, any young man of age 25 to 35 who consumes alcohol has a 12.4% chance [8] of becoming an alcoholic. These odds are terrible.

Most men in this age group would not be playing golf or tennis if these sports carried a 12.4% chance of death or lifelong serious illness. With these facts in mind, it is interesting how many in the USA ignore the dangers of social alcohol.

30% of all highway deaths are due to drunk driving [12]. The total number of drunk driving highway deaths per year is 10,265 [12] and this number is absolutely preventable *if* society makes some changes.

With this 10,265 number staring us in the face, it seems that society sort of shrugs and accepts this terrible number. This is a travesty. These deaths should absolutely not occur.

One might say, "Well, if people could just drink responsibly, there would be no problem." Unfortunately, society has tried that statement for decades and it has not worked.

Social Alcohol

This 10,265 number mentions highway alcohol related deaths. This number does not mention the alcohol related car crash disabilities, such as life changing injuries, leaving people wheel chair bound or minus and arm or leg, or with mental changes or permanent paralyses secondary to the crashes.

Of the yearly 1,070 traffic deaths in children ages 0 to 14 years, 16% involve alcohol impaired drivers. [12] For all ages, the 10,265 number for alcohol related car crash deaths is just part of the story.

Each year, there are 88,000 alcohol related deaths due to all causes, car crashes included. Each day, there are 28 people dying from alcohol related car crashes and each day there are 241 deaths due to alcohol from all causes.

This number, 241 deaths per day, is wild! It is crazy! What would we do if we had 241 deaths per day from drinking soda? Would we say, "Just drink soda responsibly?" No, we would likely ban soda.

How would we react if we had 241 deaths per day due to high school or college football? Would we tell the football athletes, "Please be careful?" Hardly. Football would be banned in a hurry.

We in the USA give alcohol a unique place of honor and immunity to criticism. The result is 88,000 deaths per year. Every one of those deaths is preventable.

54
The Ten–Year Dilemma

A person might state, "I have no problems with alcohol. I only have a couple of drinks a day and I handle it well."

The problems here are: One or two drinks daily, now, could quickly change to many more daily drinks in ten years and in ten years many good people have succumbed to the major problems with alcohol. This is the dilemma. We do not know which persons will succumb ten years from now and which persons will not. It is entirely unpredictable.

Another defect with the theory of "I can handle a couple of drinks a day" is that just one or two drinks in any human can result in behavior changes, psychological changes, motor defects and thinking difficulties. [3]

So, what if another person nearby needs urgent medical attention? How efficient will the one or two daily drinks person be? Another different problem with the one or two daily drink theory is that this habit is a daily advertisement that alcohol is really OK because the drinking person is not skunk drunk.

Many peers, adults and children alike, are vulnerable. So, the observers begin drinking and they run into problems, which can be multiple and severe.

55
Habits of Societies

Habits of societies are heavily influenced by money, advertising, public opinion and politics.

Habits of societies (large groups of people) are often influenced less by death rates.

Therefore, the habit of using alcohol is difficult to break, regardless of its death rate (mortality) or its morbidity (rate of sickness or major illness).

We are going to need more than illness and death rate statistics to change our alcohol consumption habits.

We will need other methods to influence public opinion, as mentioned later, in "Our Choices," page 136

56
Let's Try an Experiment

Let's say that you are a male. You are about 30. You live in a community that never heard of alcohol. You've actually heard of the drug alcohol, you came from a community where you knew all about it; you knew all of the facts about the drug.

Let's say that you are going to invite 100 males, all roughly in your age group, to your house for a social gathering. You are thinking about beverages. Remember, none of these men have ever heard of alcohol.

So, you have a decision to make. You need to decide whether to serve alcohol and introduce all of these 100 men to this substance, or you may decide against introducing alcohol to these 100 men.

The statistics are simple. If you introduce the drug to these men in a way that tastes good and, if they decide to become drinkers for the rest of their lives, twelve of them will become alcoholics (the actual figure is 12.4%). [56]

A significant number of the drinkers who are not addicted, will have alcohol related major events in the future, such as car crashes which cause death and other bad problems, even though they are not addicted. A percentage of them will die from their use of the substance.

Social Alcohol

If you introduce alcohol to these 100 men, the chances are good that they will introduce the drug to some others. So that could produce the domino effect, or the pebble and ripples on the lake effect. The idea could spread, and the result could be many more folks using the drug, compared to the original 100.

Now, at the beginning of the social time at your house, before you introduced the "new drug" to them, let's say that some of them questioned why you wanted to propose that they use this new drug.

You need to think in advance about how to answer that. Will it help their lives? Will it help them at work? Do you really want to introduce this agent to those who have never heard of it? It is a point to ponder.

Now, let 's say that you are 30–year old woman. Put yourself in the same situation that was used for men. 100 women, coming to your house, who have never heard of this drug called alcohol. The dangers are the same, but the numbers are different.

If you introduce this new drug to the 100 women and if they use it the rest of their lives in moderate or low amounts, the number becoming alcoholics will be about five. (Actually, the number is 4.9) [56]. And, in these daily users, who are or not alcoholic, a significant number will have major events, such as car wrecks that kill, etc. These numbers are sobering.

Now let's project into a year after the first social gathering. Same people, 12 months later. One of the guests comes up to the same host and states, "You know, you introduced us to this new material, this drug called alcohol. I tried it and did not like it, one bit. But, some of my buddies were using it and I hang out with them a lot. I thought I should use this new drug because I was fearful that they would call me a wimp or something and I wanted to be part of the crowd."

You could think, but not say, "You did not want to be called a wimp by your friends, so you decided to wimp out and do what they were doing even though you did not want to, so you became a cowardly wimp. You decided to be a lemming. You destroyed all of your self–worth and your identity. What you did was absurd."

OK. You thought that, but you did not say it. Here are words that would have been more appropriate, "Well, a lot of people do not want to be left out and a lot of people want to be accepted and be part of the crowd. But friend, be glad, because if you do not drink, as a male, you are already part of a very significant and growing crowd. 25% of all males in the USA do not drink. (For females, the figure is 37% of the population who do not drink.) [57] So, pal, if it is important to you to be 'part of the crowd' you are indeed part of a larger crowd than you may realize which does not drink."

(Later you could think, but not say, "Please get your act together buddy, and grow up, because you will be very unhappy in life if your goal is to be 'part of the crowd.'")

57
Excuses? None Needed

In her book about the advantages of not drinking [29], Annie Grace has listed several excuses people may use when in a group and they choose not to drink alcohol. These excuses are those that have come to Ms. Grace from other people and these excuses are not ones that are used by Ms. Grace.

These excuses include such statements as "I'm watching my weight" and "I'm trying to cut back" and "I'm doing an alcohol–free challenge" as well as other excuses.

She lists nine statements that nondrinkers have suggested to her to say to explain why their choice of a nonalcoholic beverage. Also, she mentions that one can order a beer in a dark bottle, get the beer, pour out the beer and replace it with water.

But hold on! Why make up phony excuses as above, which are actually lies? That is silly. Why not just say that one wants a 7-Up, or one wants ice water? What is wrong with that honest, quick approach?

Or, if the non–drinker is pressured, which by the way is very impolite of the group who wants to apply pressure, the non–drinker can laugh and say, "I will explain it to you sometime."

58

Heroin, Cocaine and Alcohol

These three drugs are addictive and they kill people.

In discussions about human behavior, a phrase is often used, "Don't even start to try heroin or cocaine, it is unwise, addiction can come rapidly, and your life can be ruined."

It is interesting that we do not as often hear that phrase about alcohol. Rather, if any advice is used, the advice may be, "When you drink alcohol, be careful and drink responsibly." Some parents may even say that they want to teach their children to drink so they can drink responsibly. This is interesting logic and is completely incorrect.

The World Health Organization reports that teens who begin alcohol before age 14 are more prone to have increased risks of alcohol abuse and dependence at later ages. [48]

It is interesting to compare the yearly death rates of these three addictive drugs. In the USA, the deaths due to cocaine are about 7,000 per year. [37] The United States yearly death rate secondary to heroin is 13,000 per year. [37] The yearly alcohol death rate is 88,000 per year.

Why does society look at these three addictive drugs differently? One reason may be that society does not take seriously the harmful effects of alcohol. Another reason could be that in the USA so much money is made on the legal use of alcohol. Massive advertisements and promotions are pushing the use of alcohol, unlike cocaine and heroin.

Social Alcohol

Expensive influential lobbying takes place in the US Congress and lobbying is effective. It would be rare for lobbyists to try to influence congress to benefit the cocaine or heroin industries. Why does society not see alcohol as dangerous as heroin and cocaine?

One reason is that alcohol is slower to destroy. Other reasons are that alcohol is heavily promoted and advertised to the U S public with the public being told that alcohol use is stylish or masculine or feminine or that alcohol is the "in" drug to consume.

59
Groupthink

If we want to participate in groupthink, this is one way of living life. That is, whatever activity other people in the group are doing, I decide to do it also.

I think: "If I do not do it, I will be an outsider and I do not want to be an outsider. It is really important to me to be one of the group. So, I will be involved in 'groupthink' which is really 'no–think.'

"If 'no–think' is my goal, I will always be a follower. Groupthink means that if all in my group are going swimming, I must do that also. If all in my group are attending a soccer game, I had better go, even though I hate soccer. If all are using marijuana, I had better join in.

"Groupthink means that I do not dare show any individualism, because if I do, the people in my group may say that I am different, and they may not like me. Groupthink means that I simply go along with the crowd. Groupthink means that I may not make a courageous decision.

"It is so important to me to be part of the group, no matter what the group is doing. With groupthink, I may be willing to endure harm to avoid criticism or rejection."

Examples of groupthink are everywhere — in science, politics, medicine, education, business and theology.

Groupthink is extremely common.

We only need to look around to see it.

60
Think the Unthinkable

Think the unthinkable and do what has not been done. Have a social gathering and do not serve alcohol. Your boss will come to your house for the social gathering. Your boss may say, "Where is the booze?" You will say, "We are not serving it tonight." You will be fearful that your boss will be critical. Well, maybe it could be that when your boss thinks it over, he/she may respect you for it.

And what about this? It could be that your boss has been considering stopping the drug herself or himself.

Could it be that if your boss sees YOU not serving the drug at some function, this could precipitate your boss to get up some courage (get his guts up, or her guts up, as my football coach used to say) and perhaps your boss could stop using and serving the drug?

What about your neighbors? Will they tease you because you served no alcohol? Maybe. They may not respect you. Who cares? YOU are the boss of your life. Don't let the neighbors run your life.

61
It Is NOT Just About You

In many a casual conversation, the statement made is, "I can use alcohol responsibly and I know I will never be an alcoholic. I can go through life this way and there will never be a problem."

Let's be careful with that statement. First, how do you know that you will go through life and never have a problem? Many people have made that statement and, some time later, a destructive problem developed — brought on by an alcohol related destructive lack of judgment, lack of self–control or uncontrolled outburst of temper.

Or alcoholism may surface. One might say, "Ridiculous, that will never happen to me."

Hold on! It has happened to hundreds of thousands of people.

A second point about this casual statement is this entire subject is not *just all about me*. Let's say that I could go through life doing moderate to minimal drinking and let's say I never did have an adverse event and I never did turn alcoholic. The point is, it isn't *just all about me*. I am influencing dozens of teenagers, pre–teens and vulnerable and fragile peers, even many adults.

Social Alcohol

By seeing me drink, I am advertising the drug to them and they assume that this drug must be good. So, I am silently giving them the green light to go ahead and drink. With that green light, some will not be able to handle the drug alcohol. They will have an alcohol related event or they will become alcoholics.

Bill Clinton has smoked cigars. It is hard to know how many per month but that does not matter. Maybe enough to bring on cancer and bad lung disease; maybe not. The point is, Bill and his cigars have advertised tobacco, with the green light effect, telling youth and vulnerable peers that tobacco is fine. Many people who follow his green light effect will not get into trouble with tobacco, but many will. He has set an example for others to follow.

If we are going to be leaders, the green light effect is there constantly.

62
Hey, Men, Get Over It!

Hey men! Hey, you softball guys, you golfers, you card players and you city league basketball players. Just get over it! You can still be a good guy, you can still be accepted, and you will not be kicked off of the team if you don't drink alcohol.

Yes, you can still be masculine, and you can still be part of the group. Sure, at first you could be harassed when your buddies see you not drinking. That is OK. If, after the game, eight of you go to have a few beers and eight of you are drinking, then one of the eight will be an alcoholic someday.

Or, after the game, if nine of you go out for some refreshments and if you are not a drinker and if eight other guys are having a few beers, one of the eight of them will be an alcoholic. Since you are not drinking, you will never be an alcoholic.

Do remember the numbers. If you do not drink, you will never be an alcoholic. If you do drink, that one in eight chance is pretty clear. Not a real pleasant number.

So, men, get over it. Yes, you can still be one of the guys if you decide not to drink. And you could get some respect, for showing that you are a thinker with something called courage.

Sometimes we call this "guts."

63

Does Alcohol Make You Courageous?

George Washington thought so. Just before a battle he followed the British practice and delivered a double portion of rum to his soldiers. On military ships today, the US Navy has a rule of no alcohol, before a battle or anytime.

Annie Grace, in her book [29] states that alcohol gives a false sense of bravado, with delayed reactions and dulled senses. Grace states that alcohol makes us less aware of our instincts, resulting in us being stupid, rather than brave.

So, George Washington was not correct to give his soldiers a double portion of rum. He was absolutely wrong. His double portion of rum was actually quite harmful to his soldiers' skill and efficiency.

Airline pilots must be brave and courageous. Airlines forbid even a trace of alcohol to be in the blood of a commercial pilot, before starting to pilot a plane. For pilots who choose to drink, there is a rule that states there must be a certain number of hours from bottle to throttle.

Surgeons must have bravery and courage to do an operation well. If a surgeon has alcohol on board in the operating room, the surgeon is ushered out of the operating room and invited to meet with a committee to discuss future actions he /she may take. Actions may include, in some cases, 6 months of rehabilitation before returning to the operating room.

64
We Doctors are Guilty

I am a doctor and I say, "We doctors are lazy and we are guilty when it comes to alcohol problems with our patients. We shrug our shoulders. Yet, the problems are vivid. We see the problems in our patients."

Many hospital admissions are related to alcohol problems [55] and we doctors shrug our shoulders. Perhaps we do not want to offend our patients, fearing that they will leave our practice and go to another doctor. And we do not want to offend our peers.

Example: If we see another doctor with a cast on his or her arm, we say, "why the cast?" But if we see a peer at a social function with loads of alcohol on board, we often say nothing. Perhaps we do not want to offend him or her. We simply do not want to bring up that subject.

It is simple to discuss a cast on the arm of a peer. It is most difficult to discuss how the peer is doing with alcohol use.

65
What Is Good for All Humanity?

When one makes a decision regarding whether he or she should use alcohol, one should simply ask the question as follows:

What does the greatest good for all of humanity?

If all of humanity uses this drug and using this drug does the greatest good, so be it. However, the evidence today is that if all of humanity consumes the drug alcohol, this is not consistent with the greatest good.

The obvious conclusion is that it does no good at all for all of humanity to consume the drug alcohol. So it would be simple if we humans voluntarily and of our own will, just stopped using it and serving it.

That is simple.

Extremely simple.

66
Politically Correct

Politically correct? Now let's see, let's look at this. What does politically correct mean? Does it mean pleasing your boss, pleasing your peers or pleasing whom?

Do you want to drink since you think that your boss wants you to drink or to increase your job security? Actually, maybe your boss does not even care what you consume, be it alcohol or non–alcohol.

Or maybe your boss will respect you more if you are not drinking. If you drink, thinking that it will increase your job security, that is odd that you use a potent, potentially habit–forming drug so you will think it will help you keep a job.

At home, is it politically correct to drink so that you can please your children, hoping that they will grow up and drink, getting the habit, so that they in the future could be in the significant percentage of drinkers who become alcoholic?

Let's see now ... politically correct?

Whom are we pleasing?

67

Prostate Cancer and Alcohol

What does alcohol have to do with prostate cancer? It is this: An estimated 26,730 men died of prostate cancer in the year 2016 in the USA. [1]

We as a society are very concerned about prostate cancer; we treat it vigorously and test for it constantly. Well, in the same year that we had 26,730 deaths from prostate cancer, we also had 88,000 deaths from alcohol.

What are we doing about those 88,000 alcohol deaths? We are encouraging people to drink.

Huge amounts of money are involved with encouraging people to drink, with many TV ads, billboard and newspaper ads and athletic event ads.

Society is going all out to stop prostate cancer and society is going all out to encourage people to drink alcohol. This seems sort of odd. But society goes where the money is and massive amounts of advertising money attracts many people to alcohol.

68
Why Do *We* Drink?

Because we are told to.
- ✓ Society tells us to
- ✓ Friends tell us to
- ✓ Advertising tells us to

So why do we drink?

We are told to.

And we dutifully follow instructions.

69

We Humans Do Things for Certain Reasons

As humans, we do not just do things. We do things for reasons.

There are many theories about why we use alcohol. One is peer approval, another is a numbing of emotional pain and another is loosening of the tongue for conversation.

Take peer approval. What? Is peer approval so important that a human would use this life–threatening drug alcohol just to be approved by our peers?

How about the numbing of emotional pain? What? Some humans need to be drugged up with this dangerous drug alcohol to combat emotional pain?

What about US Navy personnel at sea, on ships? With or without a battle at sea, there is no alcohol on U S Naval ships.

So, we on the land, living in a safe community, must have alcohol to combat emotional pain, while naval men and women at sea cannot use it? What is wrong with this picture?

On board a naval ship, emotional pain can certainly be as great or greater than the emotional pain that we land dwellers experience. How about us using other doctor approved medications and methods to combat our emotional pain?

And loosening the tongue for conversation? What? The same reasoning holds. So, are we humans so weak and insecure that we need this drug alcohol in our bodies just to talk casually with another human?

What is going on here?

What are we, a bunch of weaklings, to need this drug alcohol so often?

70
What's in Our House?

If we have the polio virus in our house and our child dies of polio, it's a tragedy. We do everything we can to eradicate the polio virus. If we have bacteria in our house and our child dies of meningitis from the bacteria, it is a tragedy. We do all that we can to eradicate bacteria.

Now, let's say that our child dies of an alcohol related incident. It is a tragedy. What do we do about the alcohol? Do we leave it in our house? Why? Because it is stylish to leave it in our house? And, when people come over, we're expected to serve it. Style is so very important ... right?

Now ... if we kept a loaded gun in our house and a child had a terrible accident as a result, we might remove the gun. But ... what about removing alcohol? Well ... keeping the drug alcohol in the house with easy availability is more acceptable than keeping a loaded gun available. We humans often do what is stylish, no matter what the result may be.

71
It Is Part of Our Society?

When we look at death, heartache and disability, all resulting from alcohol, a solution is simple. The solution is: Do not consume the drug. Do not consume it and do not sell it.

The solution is quite simple and direct. But many community leaders might say that this drug is entrenched in our society; it is a source of revenue and a source of employment. These leaders might say that the answer is to simply control the drug, educate the public and use the drug in moderation.

That advice from leaders may sound good, but the quick reply to that theory is that the approach they suggest has not ever worked and it is not working now. That theory has been tried for decades and it does not work.

That theory was used regarding slavery. Slavery was entrenched in our society and it was a source of great economic prosperity. It was said, "Slavery is an economic force we are used to, so let's keep it and use it in moderation."

But, with slavery, we finally had to pay the price and we stopped using it. The slavery "source of revenue" went away and our country survived.

Similarly, we should stop using alcohol. That is the answer.

72
New Ideas

Now, let's discuss ideas. Let's look back a little in history. Let's say 60 years before the Civil War, in a village about 80 miles south of Atlanta.

What about this — what if a writer proposed an idea that slavery should be obliterated? Many would have laughed and many would have ridiculed the writer stating that it just did not make any sense. Slavery was part of our nation and, besides, it was part of our economy.

Let's consider another idea — the idea of women's suffrage. What if someone proposed, 100 years before women's suffrage became part of our nation's law, that women be allowed to vote? Well, it just did not make sense. We weren't doing that, and it just was not part of our society.

Another idea — the idea of dueling. In the year 1800, when dueling was a gentlemanly thing to do, what if a gentleman who was challenged to a duel stated that this was not a reasonable and correct way to solve an argument? He would have been considered a coward, made a social outcast and, perhaps, forced into bankruptcy. Society stated that dueling was the way to solve certain disputes.

Public punishment, in the town square, often with the guilty person in locks, was cruel and destructive; now eliminated. In the US military, in the past, flogging was a form of discipline that has now gone by the wayside.

What about the idea of someone objecting to witchcraft trials in Massachusetts around the year 1790? Any person questioning the witchcraft trials may have been ostracized, indeed. Witchcraft was accepted to be present and those accused of it were punished — quite severely, in fact.

Actually, when something is accepted in society and a person proposes that this "something" that is accepted be changed, different reactions come forth. Some reactions are those of ridicule, some are those of ignoring, some state that the new idea simply is not economically feasible, and some accuse the new idea of being absurd.

Well, here is a new idea: social alcohol really is not needed. Some will say that this new idea certainly is not economically feasible. Look how many people depend on this drug for their livelihood. Marketers, advertisers, manufacturers, distributors and consumers make up a huge amount of money changing hands, all for the use of this drug.

Well, this could be changed, and our society could survive. Our society has always survived when new ideas have been carried out.

73

Opioid Deaths and Alcohol Deaths

Recently, the USA has had a vigorous campaign to cut down on opioid deaths which numbered over 42,000 in 2016. [58] However, opioids are legitimate pain killers and there are very acceptable indications for their use.

It is good that authorities encourage the correct use of these medications and, if opioids are not used correctly, then we have horrible results, such as addiction and deaths.

These 42,000 deaths in just one year are tragedies. The manufacture and sale of prescription opioids brings very little tax revenue into governments and legitimate opioid sales do little to increase numbers in our country's workforce. So, if prescription opioid consumption is decreased, there would be not much popular resistance in the USA except for those profiting from the opioid business.

Conversely, it is interesting to see that there is little press and not much attention paid to the 88,000 alcohol related USA deaths per year, this number remaining pretty constant, year after year.

In the last year I have not read one article in the lay press showing concern about the 88,000 alcohol deaths per year, while the mainstream media have had many presentations about the tragic nature of opioid deaths which are only a fraction of the alcohol deaths.

Also, it is interesting that alcohol manufacture and sales provide many jobs for our economy and tax revenues from alcohol are very large. One wonders if these factors explain why the leaders of our country have not embarked on a vigorous program to decrease alcohol related deaths.

One way to decrease alcohol deaths is to decrease consumption. If the country's leaders embarked on a vigorous campaign to decrease consumption, big alcohol financial interests would likely be very displeased.

So, our country remains silent about the status quo and quietly accepts the 88,000 alcohol deaths per year.

Michael Bloomberg, the former mayor of New York City, has spent millions of dollars promoting campaigns to decrease and hopefully cease the use of tobacco. [58] One could speculate on the same approach to alcohol use. It would cost millions of dollars and the alcohol industry would, of course, fight any campaign to decrease alcohol use. But, if rich benefactors approached the subject, progress could result.

The Bloomberg Initiative to combat tobacco use was boosted when the Bill and Melinda Gates Foundation teamed up with Bloomberg. [58] Decreased tobacco usage resulted.

Similarly, if several rich leaders worked together on alcohol usage, public opinion could be changed, and alcohol use could plummet. This is not out of the question by any means.

We just have not tried it yet.

74
AIDS Deaths and Alcohol Deaths

In the United States, for the last year reported [59] the number of deaths attributed directly to HIV AIDS was 6,721.

For the last year reported, the number of alcohol related deaths was 88,000.

Millions of dollars are being spent yearly to find ways to treat and prevent AIDS. Scientists are performing excellent, complex research projects to help prevent the deaths from AIDS and to help prevent the AIDS virus from starting in a person.

One wonders why, in the USA, we do not spend millions to decrease the 88,000 yearly deaths from alcohol.

75
Comparisons

In the horrible tragedy of 9–11–2001, about 3,000 people died. Each year 88,000 people die with alcohol related problems.

After the 9–11 tragedy, banner headlines were prominent. The utter horror of it all was more than terrible. Lives were changed forever after 9–11 and 9–11 changed our country's way of living.

What about the 88,000 deaths each year from alcohol? Each year alcohol kills 29 times the number of deaths from 9–11.

We humans scarcely blink an eye. This figure may not even be in the newspaper. We pay little or no attention to this tragedy.

76

Cars

If each of us, upon starting to drive, would learn that driving a car would bring to all males a 12% death rate or serious injury rate, we would be sobered.

Similarly, if all ladies, upon starting to drive, knew that they would have a 4.9% chance of death or serious injury, this would be frightening.

This knowledge would make all of us very concerned about our driving. Well, we could compare driving cars to consuming alcohol. Every young man or young woman who starts using alcohol, even conservatively at age 21, can face pretty grim statistics.

Those statistics are that 12.4% of all men who begin drinking alcohol will be addicted in future years and 4.9% of all women who consume alcohol will be addicted in the future. These numbers are terrible but true.

If we applied these unfortunate numbers to driving cars, we would likely demand some changes. We should also be demanding changes relating to alcohol's dangers.

77

A Culture of Minimal Expectations

Interesting phrase — "A culture of minimal expectations." One wonders if that is what we have in the U S A. Does this phrase apply to us as we often ignore the horrible results of alcohol use?

During World War II, we did not have that culture of minimal expectations —we went all out to win that war. We sacrificed to win that war.

We often have that culture of minimal expectations as we hear about horrible deaths and disability due to alcohol. It may be that we shrug our shoulders and change our thinking to something else.

If we Americans do not expect a change, we will not get a change. Indeed, we often are participating in a culture of minimal expectations.

78
Relative Opinions

Frank Bruno [60] of the New York Times, states that in the USA, in our hypercritical public discussions about substance abuse, drinking often gets a pass. That is because it is legal and widely used as a sociable pastime. But, Bruni states, "Alcohol kills far more people than powders, capsules and vials." Bruni reports that about one third of the US population is either addicted to alcohol or binge drinks dangerously.

He states that if we Americans are going to discuss our drug problems with any honesty, then we should not "leave alcohol out of the picture."

Bruni makes a good point. At many government and large corporate functions, alcohol flows quite freely. But if a leader or participant in one of those functions used marijuana during the meeting, in a state that has legalized marijuana, what number of eyebrows would be raised? What would the press say?

This is odd because marijuana kills no one and alcohol kills 88,000 US humans per year. We Americans have different reasoning methods for different substances. Huge amounts of money are spent in this country to promote the alcohol industry. This is a fast train that has much momentum. Many leaders who know of alcohol's great problems simply do not want to tackle the problem.

They would rather work on opioids with the 2015 mortality rate from opioids of 42,000. This figure includes deaths from prescription opioids, heroin and fentanyl.

It is easy to attack opioids. No tax revenue is brought in from opioids while alcohol brings large incomes into many parts of our country.

We attack what is popular to attack.

It is not popular to attack alcohol because alcohol often is where the money is.

79

If You Always Do What You Always Did

A rancher in the southwest was discussing ways to improve profits on his land. He was a thinker and a planner, as well as an honest businessman. While talking to a group of other ranchers, he made a statement that later was often repeated. He said, "If you always do what you did, you will always get what you got."

Grammatically that may not be the most beautiful sentence, but it applies to life and it applies to alcohol. If we humans continue to do what we have always done, we will continue to get our 88,000 deaths per year as well as the added suffering which is difficult to measure.

The segments of our society who are making a lot of money on alcohol would certainly agree with the rancher's statement. Those who are making a lot of money on this drug simply love our current situation. Because of the profits involved, many elements in our country are not worried about the deaths per year or the yearly suffering from this drug.

80
Ladies, Get Over It!

Ladies, and this means ladies and girls of all ages, please think this over very carefully ...

Let's say that you are part of a group of twenty of your peers, including you. You walk in and you see that the other 19 are all drinking something alcoholic. You can join the others, be part of the gang and order a similar drink. That way you won't be different.

But why not be different? When you join the group, if you decide to be one of the twenty ladies using alcohol, one of you will become an alcoholic someday — that's a proven fact. [8] One out of twenty ... that is 5% of the ladies in this room will become an alcoholic. And your decision is telling the others, "It is fine to use this drug."

Does it take courage to make the decision to drink something alcoholic with the others? Of course not. It takes not one bit of courage to be part of the group.

Why not try another approach? When you join the group, if you decide not to drink alcohol, then you become one of the group who will not become an alcoholic. And your decision is telling the others, "It is fine to not use this drug and I can still have a great time."

So how about just ordering a soft drink or water? Your peers may tease you and give you a hard time, but some will also admire you.

Social Alcohol

In that group of twenty ladies, it is very likely that at least one or two might be an alcoholic or on the road to becoming an alcoholic. But if they watch you and see the courage you are showing, it might give them the courage to not drink anymore alcohol this time.

What if your boss is in this group of twenty women and she loves to drink? Please don't think you have to drink to please your boss. Just get over it. Who knows? Your boss might be looking for someone in the group who is strong enough to take a different path, such as not drinking.

There may also be several others in the group who are very vulnerable and looking for someone who is not drinking. Maybe they, or your boss, want to begin their own non–drinking program, something that may have been their goal for a long time. Yes, with your actions, you can be a silent, encouraging person to your boss and others.

If people give you a hard time about your not drinking, you know they are being rude. Just ignore it, give them a gracious, warm, genuine smile, and say, "I'm a 7–Up person." Then laugh and change the subject.

Avoid saying or hinting anything that sounds like you are being judgmental — people resent that. And, when you change the subject, you might ask the person something about themselves. People love to talk about their own lives.

Remember the chapter in this book that quotes Annie Grace? (page 90) She lists, "Excuses That People Use in Order Not to Drink." The excuses that Annie Grace quotes are not hers but are the excuses of others. They are phony, ridiculous and absurd.

Oh yes, the title of this chapter states, "Ladies Get Over It!" This means ladies of all ages (teens to age 99) and lifestyles. Yes, try it and you will find that it is, indeed, easier than you think, to "get over it."

You will be glad that you did.

And oh yes. Do you know who else will profit from your decision? Your husband or partner, your children, your extended family and many more, both women and men.

You can count on it.

81
What's Wrong with Being Extreme?

You may have heard the statement, "Oh, he or she is an extremist" or "Don't be an extremist." Somewhere along the line in our society, we have instilled the idea that it is somehow incorrect to be extreme. We have stated in so many words that it is correct to be a moderate and it is best to be in the middle of the road on many subjects.

Why NOT be an extremist on some subjects? Christopher Columbus was an extremist. Simmelweiss was definitely accused of being an extremist when, as a doctor in Vienna in 1850, he urged all doctors in the hospital to wash their hands before caring for patients.

He was ridiculed, chastised and belittled because of his "extreme" views. Doctors were gentlemen, he was told and gentlemen never washed their hands. When the doctors did begin to wash their hands, the infection and death rates plummeted. Simmelweiss was correct.

Another "extreme" individual was Dr. Reginald Fitz, in Boston in 1886. He suggested that some patients, with fever and pain in the right lower abdomen and other symptoms, might need to have their appendix removed.

This was a new and "extreme" idea. Not only was he branded as extreme, he was almost dismissed from the prestigious Boston Medical Society because his suggestion of removing the appendix had never been considered before.

British surgeon Dr. Joseph Lister, in the mid 1800's, revolutionized surgical thinking when he suggested that surgical instruments should be sterile, and surgeons should wear sterile attire and sterile gloves.

American surgeons ignored Lister, scoffing at his extreme ideas, when they were caring for President Garfield, who had a gunshot wound in 1881.

As they cared for President Garfield, they used dirty instruments and unclean hands. The bullet wound would not have killed Garfield because the bullet was lodged in a harmless location. Death came due to massive, generalized infection, due to the doctors not using sterile technique as they cared for him.

Well ...here is an "extreme" idea: Society does not really need social alcohol and society would be better off without it.

An extreme idea? Depends on your point of view.

Would the idea be extreme if it saved 88,000 lives per year? The 88,000 people who lived might say that the idea was not extreme at all. Their families and loved ones might agree.

82

Times Change and Needs Change

When we look at history, times change and needs change. Buggy whips, the horse and buggy, the steam railroad locomotive, the covered wagon and the manual typewriter are just about all gone.

History is full of examples of things or habits that appeared to be needed. Then the realization came that their usefulness or their supposed need had ceased.

This can be the story with social alcohol. We have thought it has been necessary, needed and a part of a "healthy social life". Now we know that social alcohol plays no useful role.

Society realized that the covered wagon was simply not needed anymore; therefore, it faded out of usage in a practical society.

The horse and buggy were replaced by other types of transportation such as the steam locomotive in some cases and the internal combustion engine in other cases.

However, society has been using social alcohol for some time. We should now realize that we do not need it any more.

We can easily phase it out simply by realizing it is not needed and we should realize that we all will be better off without it.

The way to institute this change is not by civil law. The way to achieve the change is simply to realize that consuming social alcohol potentially causes great harm. Therefore, we should just stop using it.

The automobile was a good replacement for the horse and buggy. A good replacement for social alcohol would be healthy and positive lives that do not depend on social alcohol.

83
Civilization

Gandhi was once asked, "What do you think of Western Civilization?" His reply was, "I think it would be a good idea."

One might ask a similar question, "What do you think of the world's civilization?" The answer could be, "I think it would be a good idea."

When one ponders these questions and the potential answers, one must think of habits that humans engage in today — slavery, the attractions to drugs and the glorification of drugs such as alcohol, tobacco, heroin and others.

Indeed, if we are going to have a civilized society, why do we need to honor alcohol and other substances which bring such great harm? We humans do things that destroy ourselves, over and over and over.

Somehow, we think that is "the thing to do."

84
Culture Changes

Cultures can be changed. Our country changed away from slavery. The tobacco culture in our country is changing, slowly but surely. Women were not allowed to vote in the USA until fairly recently and that culture has undergone a 100% change. Witch hunts and witch killings in this country were a standard part of our culture and that culture has changed.

The culture of clothing styles changes all the time. Can we imagine a US president today wearing a black stove pipe hat, as yesterday's presidents did? In our country, it was common for many women to dip snuff and smoke pipes. Today fewer women smoke pipes and dip snuff compared to yesteryear.

The culture of communication changes all the time. For example, in the late nineteenth century, Alexander Graham Bell introduced the telephone at an inventor's convention in Philadelphia. As different scientists witnessed the human voice being carried from one room to another, one scientist remarked, "Interesting invention, but of what use will it ever be?"

What an amazing change the telephone made in our culture! Think of the massive cultural change because computers now are commonplace. Our grandparents certainly did not have computers.

Social Alcohol

What about the culture of alcohol? Can that culture be changed? Of course, it can! The pros and cons are obvious. The pros are that, if we eliminate beverage alcohol from our society, we would have a healthier society and we would eliminate 88,000 deaths per year. Also, we would eliminate alcohol's morbidity and heartache.

The cons of eliminating alcohol are, well, the cons are we people just may not want to change. Maybe we thinking humans want to just leave it like it is. Maybe we just think that the status quo is permanent. Maybe we do not want to fight the system. We do not want to appear unpopular. Alcohol brings in much in the way of tax revenue.

We can think of many reasons to not make any changes whatsoever.

85
Logic

Think about logic. If, in America, there is ever going to be a movement that will decrease alcohol's mortality and morbidity, the movement will be fueled by logic. Logic is a strong talking point.

Logic is a talking point that adds fuel to the idea of decreasing alcohol's mortality and morbidity. Logic will need to combat industry, since logic does not make money for industry.

Logic does not have Madison Avenue on its side and logic makes no money for the manufacturers, marketers and distributors of alcohol.

86
Cups of Tea

There are phrases, often used such as, "that's my cup of tea" or "that is just not my cup of tea." These statements are legitimate, honest and good. They can apply to anything. They can apply to food choices, how we spend our time and how and why we do anything.

Up to now, our country has made, silently, a very honest and subtle statement:

In the USA, we citizens feel that it is just not our cup of tea to do anything about the 88,000 alcohol related deaths per year and it is not our cup of tea to address the horrible yearly morbidity from alcohol.

We know that alcohol inspired beatings of children and wives occur daily and some alcohol related car crashes result in life changing physical defects such as permanent paralyses of arms and legs. But it is not our cup of tea to take measures to change these numbers.

Actually, we do not care much about the numbers and we may decide to stay with the status quo, in that we don't feel any pressure from peers or family to make any changes.

87

Crazy?

Are some of the ideas in this book crazy? Some might say so. Throughout history many new ideas have been branded as crazy.

Branch Rickey was told he was crazy for hiring Jackie Robinson, the first African American to play major league baseball. Of course, his decision was correct.

In England, the idea that slavery could be abolished was branded as crazy.

Are some of the ideas in this book crazy? Not at all. They are simply new ideas. Some segments of the population do not like new ideas. Some say it is better to live with the status quo.

The status quo is causing 88,000 deaths per year in the USA. That number of yearly deaths is a horrible price to pay for the luxury of not disturbing the status quo.

Maintaining and accepting the status quo always comes with a high price and it is always paid by you and me.

88
CDC Research and Advice

The Center for Disease Control and Prevention (CDC) has done intensive research on alcohol related problems in this country. The CDC is a large organization doing excellent research, staffed by many scientists, funded by the federal government. The CDC has issued four suggestions to approach the alcohol problem. [61]

1.   Increase tax on alcohol

2.   Decrease outlet density

> This means that communities should decrease the numbers of retailers selling alcohol, resulting in fewer retailers per square mile.

> Example: If in the past, there were two alcohol retailers in one block, the change would result in one retailer in that block.

> Research has shown that the more alcohol retailers in given areas, the greater the incidence of violence in those areas. [62] [63]

3.   Decrease the days and hours of alcohol sales.

4.   Hold alcohol retailers liable for injuries or damage done by their intoxicated or underage customers.

These CDC suggestions look satisfactory on paper, but it is obvious that they would be very difficult to implement in small or large communities and increasing the tax might result in more illegal alcohol imports and sales.

All four suggestions could be objected to by retailers and alcohol manufacturers, in that potential decreases in consumption could result in large financial losses for retailers, manufacturers and people dependent on the alcohol industry for making a living.

All four suggestions would be very difficult to carry out, but we must not give up on them.

Actually, all four suggestions are not at all practical. I believe that, rather than "say nothing" about the 88,000 deaths per year from alcohol, the U. S. Government felt that they had to "make some type of a positive statement" to address this tragedy.

Consequently, their four suggestions are lame ones, carrying minimal practical value. If any of the four suggestions were tried, alcohol retailers would have decreased profits with the resulting decreased tax revenue flow to different levels of local and state government.

The CDC has protected its image so that, if challenged, they can say, "Well we issued four suggestions and Americans did not follow our advice."

89
What We Need

- ✓ We need a few people who can invite people over to their houses and **not** say, "I don't want to offend my boss who is coming over because my boss is a guest, you know, and my boss likes alcohol. I really don't need alcohol myself, but I want to serve alcohol, so my boss will be comfortable."

- ✓ I, plus a few others, need to say that stopping the use of alcohol is an idea whose time has come. There are really no negatives to this concept.

- ✓ We need to focus on the mindset of Rosa Parks who, in 1955, decided that the mindset that "everybody accepted" where people with different skin colors sat on buses was wrong.

Rosa Parks challenged this, and this paradigm began to change because of one person who made the challenge. She is to be congratulated, admired and respected and we need more individuals now to challenge the paradigm that "social alcohol is accepted and is harmless."

✓ We need to approach the leaders of our churches and communities and say, "Hey, of course you think what you are doing is stylish, your minimal use of alcohol socially, but remember that you are an example. Your minimal use of alcohol tells all in your group or your parish that alcohol is fine. This opens the door for others to start their minimal use of alcohol which later can work rapidly into a situation which is not so minimal."

Yes, we need to talk to our church and other leaders and ask them to think it over. We need to say, "In the long run, is it worth it?"

✓ We need to realize that if changes are made in alcohol consumption in the USA, this will be a challenge because of the massive financial and corporate pressures involved to encourage everyone — yes, everyone, to drink.

90
Our Choices

- ✓ We could do nothing and live with the status quo.
- ✓ We could strive to make it cool and stylish to not drink. This could spread like wildfire and this could be very effective in small and large communities. But this would take courage.

At first it would mean taking a lot of criticism. Later it would catch on as the neat thing to do. All age groups could perform this very easily. This would require no financial investment.

This method could be especially challenging for large, fund raising dinners, the latter of which capitalize on large alcohol consumption to be successful.

Here is how this works: Let's say that a large charity wants to make a lot of money. At the dinner, each guest obtains a ticket for one or two free drinks. Also, wine is served liberally to each dinner guest without charge.

As the dinner progresses, each guest can consume a lot of alcohol, some being free to the consumer. Then, each guest can fill out a card with their pledge — a promised donation to the charity. The more alcohol that is served, the greater the pledges and gifts. If no alcohol is served, the total money pledged is much less. [64] [65]

✓ We could enlist big money. Real big money from sources like Gates, Buffet, Bloomberg and many others. These big money sources could pay for TV ads reminding us that we can have more fun without alcohol and that there is no safe level of alcohol consumption.

Then, we would need to have enough money, real big money, to combat the powerful lobbies and other methods of the alcohol industry. We would have to be aware that the alcohol industry loves to have scientists and doctors on various boards of directors. These board members are encouraged to do research or sponsor research set up in ways to minimize the dangers of alcohol. In past years, these board members tried to fund research to say that alcohol has health benefits.

Currently the World Health Organization, along with the United Kingdom, remind us that there are no health benefits to alcohol.

In the United States Dietary Guidelines, published by the US Government, the concept that small amounts of daily alcohol could be beneficial to health, has been eliminated.

✓ Whatever we do, if we do anything at all, we must remember that to make changes can be very difficult. Many United States citizens make big, big money on alcohol.

It was difficult to eliminate slavery in the USA and now that slavery is over, we have eliminated the death rate from slavery. We made a difficult change when we made women's suffrage possible.

Social Alcohol

We were courageous enough to fight against horrible powers in WWII and we eliminated the terrible consequences awaiting us, had we not fought. We have declared that tobacco has no health benefits and, despite massive lobbying from big tobacco, progress is being made regarding that drug's death rate.

Alcohol consumption can be a tough nut to crack but the task is before us. We can approach it or ignore it. Ignoring it is easiest.

When we ignore it, people keep dying, every day. Doing nothing means people keep dying, every day.

These deaths are absolutely preventable.

91
We Can Do Different Things

On the subject of alcohol, we can do different things. One approach is to simply do what we have been doing. As Albert Einstein said, "We cannot solve our problems with the same thinking that we used when we caused them."

That means that if we continue to do the same things about alcohol that we have always done, we will continue to get over 1500 alcohol related deaths on college campuses, plus about 88,000 deaths per year, countrywide, due to the drug.

Those 88,000 deaths annually are equal to 176 jumbo jets crashing in one year, killing all passengers. We as a society would not put up with that.

Another approach would be to use a 1–month plan. What is the 1–month plan? The plan means that one family would consume no alcohol for one month. Simple and not expensive.

During that 1–month period, no family member would be involved in drunkenness and no family member would be responsible for an alcohol related car crash. No family member would be involved in alcohol related domestic violence.

Idealistic? No, not really. It could easily be done. Stylish to have one month without alcohol? That depends on who we are trying to impress.

Social Alcohol

Effective? 100% effective, except for those outside of your family who might crash into your vehicle.

What are our other choices? There are several. Like a 2–month plan or a 5–month plan or a lifetime plan.

Mark Twain was right when he said, "If you do what you've always done, you'll get what you've always got." [66]

92
Sexy Subjects

If there is a trend to avoid beverage alcohol, some might say that avoiding alcohol is just not sexy. But wait. Avoiding alcohol can be made to be sexy.

It can be made sexy by cool people on college campuses avoiding the drug and it can be made sexy by cool people in business avoiding alcohol.

Avoidance of alcohol is like a style. If it is stylish to avoid tobacco, many human lemmings avoid tobacco. If it is stylish to use tobacco, many human lemmings use tobacco.

It is the same process with alcohol. If it is stylish to use it and if everybody else is doing it, by golly, some human lemmings get into lock step and use it just like others at the party. Actually, our human logic can be quite straightforward and easy.

If everyone else in the room is drinking, this might guide behavior for lemmings.

It is so easy to be a human lemming and drink with the rest of the group.

93
Why Do You Drink?

Do you drink because it helps you as a person?

Do you drink because it helps your family?

Do you drink because it helps your country?

Do you drink because it helps the world?

Think it over.

94
Dangers of Different Drugs

In Britain, a research project was done by Britain's Center for Crime and Justice Studies and the results were published in the British medical journal Lancet. [5] The researchers evaluated different substances, including alcohol, cocaine, heroin, ecstasy, and marijuana, ranking them based on how destructive they are to the individual who takes them, and to society as a whole.

The scientists analyzed how addictive a drug is, and how the drug harms the human body in addition to other criteria, such as environmental damage caused by the drug, its role in breaking up families and its economic costs, such as health care, social services, and prison expenses.

Heroin, crack cocaine, and methamphetamine, or crystal meth, were the most lethal to individuals. When considering their wider social effects, alcohol, heroin, and crack cocaine were the deadliest. Overall, alcohol's dangers outranked all other substances with its destructive effects, followed by heroin and crack cocaine.

The dangers of marijuana, ecstasy and LSD scored far lower with their destructive effects. The study concluded that alcohol scored so high with its destruction because, they said, it is so widely used and has such devastating consequences not only for drinkers but for those around them.

Social Alcohol

After this study was published, Dr. Wim van den Brink commented on the results and his comments were published in the same journal. [67] He said, "What governments decide is illegal is not always based on science. Considerations about taxation and revenue, like those garnered from the alcohol and tobacco industries, may influence decisions about which substances to regulate or outlaw. Legal drugs cause huge amounts of damage."

I feel that these conclusions about substances in Britain no doubt apply to substances in the USA. I feel that taxation and revenue are parts of the considerations of governments about alcohol. Alcohol can be a huge money maker to society, and I feel that this is why governments do not want to touch the alcohol problem; they prefer to leave the alcohol problem alone.

Even though alcohol kills more than any other drug except tobacco, governments do not want to meddle with the income that alcohol brings in.

95
In Conclusion

As this book is completed, American society continues to face the deaths of 88,000 men, women and children each year, plus countless more lives damaged or ruined, from proven alcohol related cancer, violence, alcoholism and more.

While it is certain that there is, and will be, more research, you've read this book and you know the result — alcohol is bad for humans; it kills them.

Now it is up to each one of us to make a decision:

Will we continue to ignore the facts?

OR

Will we join together to build a climate of change that will reduce or even eliminate social alcohol?

More Detailed Definitions

Alcoholism definition: Many reliable, respected organizations have provided definitions of alcoholism and all are reasonable, while the wordings may differ somewhat. Some examples:

The Diagnostic and Statistical Manual of Mental Disorders, 5th Edition, [56] published by the American Psychiatric Association, states: An Alcohol Use Disorder is a pattern of problematic alcohol use, as manifested by at least two of the following, within a 12−month period:

1. Alcohol is taken in larger amounts or over a longer period than was intended.

2. Persistent desire or unsuccessful effort to control or cut down on alcohol use.

3. A great deal of time is spent in activities to obtain alcohol, use alcohol, or recover from its effects.

4. Craving or a strong urge to use alcohol.

5. Alcohol use is resulting in a failure to fulfill obligations at work, school, or home.

6. Continued alcohol use despite interpersonal problems caused by alcohol use.

7. Important personal activities are given up because of alcohol use.

8. Alcohol use when it is physically hazardous.

9. Alcohol use continues despite knowledge of a personal problem that has been caused or exacerbated by alcohol.

10. Tolerance, as shown by the need of increasing amounts of alcohol to achieve the desired effect.
11. Withdrawal symptoms appear upon stopping alcohol.

The World Health Organization (WHO) [3] defines alcoholism (also known as alcohol dependence) as a cluster of symptoms that develop after repeated alcohol use, including a strong desire to consume alcohol, difficulty in controlling its use, resulting in harmful consequences, increased tolerance and sometimes a withdrawal state.

The Mayo Clinic [47] states that alcoholism and alcohol use disorder are the same, both defined as having problems controlling drinking, being preoccupied with alcohol, continued use of alcohol even when it causes problems, needing to drink more to get the same effect and possibly having withdrawal symptoms.

The National Council on Alcohol and Drug Dependence (NCADD) and the American Society of Addiction Medicine (ASAM) provide similar definitions, that is: Alcohol abuse equals alcohol dependence, equals alcoholism, equals alcohol use disorder. This is a condition, often progressive and fatal, with impaired control over drinking, preoccupation with the drug alcohol, use of alcohol despite future consequences, plus thinking abnormalities, most often, denial. The person's drinking causes distress or harm to self or others.

Social Alcohol

Many other organizations (such as the American Medical Association) and multiple publications give reasonable definitions of alcoholism (alcohol use disorder) and all will not be printed here. All convey very similar definitions. There is no laboratory test to confirm or deny alcoholism.

Bibliography

[1] "United States Cancer Statistics: 1999–2013 Incidence and Mortality Web–Based Report," U.S. Cancer Statistics Working Group, 2016.

[2] *CDC Bulletin,* May 2017.

[3] Goldman-Cecil, Textbook of Medicine, 25th ed., vol. 1, Philadelphia, 2016, p. 150.

[4] K. LoConte, A. Brewster and et al, "Alcohol and cancer: a statement of The American Society of Clinical Oncology," *Journal of Clinical Oncology,* Nov 2017.

[5] L. King, L. Phillips and D. Nutt, "Drug harms in the UK: a multicriteria decision analysis," *Lancet,* vol. 376, pp. 1558-1565, Nov 2010.

[6] E. Schultz, "Ad Age," Jun 2017. [Online]. Available: http://adage.com/article/cmo-strategy/nfl-lifts-liquor-ad-ban-putting-pressure-beer/309256/.

[7] *World Health Organization Bulletin,* Jun 2017.

[8] Diagnostic and Statistical Manual of Mental Disorders, 5th ed., Arlington, VA: American Psychiatric Assn, 2013, p. 493.

[9] S. Chaudhuri, "Drink makers battle loss of health halo," *Wall St. J.,* 22 Aug 2016.

[10] A. Klatsky, G. Friedman and A. Siegelaub, "Alcohol consumption before mycardial infarction," *Ann. Intern. Med.,* vol. 81, p. 294–301, 1974.

[11] M. Cheng, *US News & World Report,* 8 Jan 2016.

[12] "Impaired driving: get the facts," *CDC Bulletin,* p. 1, Apr 2016.

[13] A. McTiernan, "One alcoholic drink a day increases breast cancer risk," American Institute of Cancer Research, May 2017.

[14] T. Chikritchs, K. Fillmore and T. Stockwell, "A healthy dose of skepticism: four good reasons to think again about protective effects of alcohol on coronary heart disease," *Drug Alcohol Rev.,* no. 4, p. 441–4, 28 Jul 2009.

[15] M. Holmes, C. Dale, L. Zuccolo and et al, "Association between alcohol and cardiovascular disease: Mendeliau randomisation," *BMJ*, p. 349, Jul 2014.

[16] K. Fillmore, T. Stockwell and et al, "Moderate alcohol use and mortality: systemic error in studies," *Annals of Epidemiology - Supplement*, vol. 17, no. 5, p. 516–523, May 2007.

[17] C. Knott, N. Coombs, E. Stamatikis and J. Biddulph, "All cause mortality and age specific alcohol guidelines: pooled analyses of 10 population based cohorts," *BMJ*, vol. 350: 384, Feb 2015.

[18] S. Andre'asson, T. Chikritzhs, F. Dangardt and et al, "Evidence about health effects of alcohol consumption: reasons for skepticism and public health implications," *Alcohol and Society*, 2014.

[19] M. Daube, "Alcohol's evaporating health benefits: industry lobbying and promotion are rife and unchecked by governments," *BMJ*, p. 350, Feb 2015.

[20] J. Zhao, T. Stockwell, A. Roemer and T. Naimi, "Alcohol consumption and mortality from coronary disease: a meta–analysis," *J Stud Alcohol Drugs*, vol. 78(3), p. 375–386, May 2017.

[21] T. Naimi, T. Stockwell and et al, "Selection bias and relationships between alcohol use and mortality," *Addiction*, vol. 112(2), p. 220–221, Feb 2017.

[22] T. Naimi, D. Brown, R. Brewer and et al, "Cardiovascular risk factors and confounders among non–drinking and moderate drinking U.S. adults," *Am J Prev Med*, vol. 28(4), p. 369–373, May 2005.

[23] R. Rabin, "Alcohol's good for you? some scientists doubt it.," *New York Times*, p. D1, 15 Jun 2007.

[24] M. Cheng, "Drinking alcohol regularly boosts cancer risk: UK officials," 8 January 2016. [Online]. Available: https://www.ctvnews.ca/health/drinking-alcohol-regularly-boosts-cancer-risk-uk-officials-1.2729539.

[25] T. Stockwell, T. Chikritzhs, T. Naimi and J. Zhao, "ISFAR doth protest too much: an attempt from industry sympathizers to marginalize scientific skepticism about alcohol's hypothesized health benefits?," *J Stud Alcohol Drugs,* vol. 77(5), pp. 839-841, Sep 2016.

[26] M. Roerecke, "Cardioprotective association of alcohol consumption: a review and meta-analysis," *Addiction,* vol. 107, no. 7, pp. 1246-1260, Jul 2012.

[27] A. Klatsky, "Alcohol and cardiovascular disease: where do we stand?," *Journal of Internal Medicine,* vol. 278, no. 3, pp. 238-250, Sep 2015.

[28] "To drink or not to drink," *Mayo Clinic Health Letter,* pp. 4-5, Mar 2016.

[29] A. Grace, This Naked Mind — Control Alcohol, Find Freedom, Discover Happiness, and Change Your Life, ASPN Publications, 2015.

[30] R. Hingson and E. Weitzman, "Magnitude of and trends in alcohol–related mortality and morbidity among U.S. college students ages 18–24, 1998–2005," *Journal of Studies on Alcohol and Drugs,* (Suppl. 16) Dec 2009.

[31] R. Hingson, T. Heeren, M. Winter and et al, "Magnitude of alcohol–related mortality and morbidity among U.S. college students ages 18–24; changes from 1998 to 2001," *Annual Review of Public Health,* vol. 26, p. 259–279, 2005.

[32] C. Blanco, M. Okuda, C. Wright and et al, "Mental health of college students and their non–college–attending–peers: results from national epidemiologic study on alcohol and related conditions," *Arch Gen Psych,* vol. 65(12), p. 1429–1437, 2008.

[33] H. Wechsler, G. Dowdall, G. Maenner and et al, "Changes in binge drinking and related problems among American college students between 1993 and 1997: Results of the Harvard School of Public Health College Alcohol Study," *J Am Coll Health,* vol. 47(2), p. 57–68, 1998.

[34] K. Reilly, "Why banning hard alcohol on college campuses may not be the answer," *Time,* Aug 2016.

[35] H. Whiteman, "Nothing to smile about: Asia's deadly addiction to betel nuts," CNN News, 5 Nov 2013.

[36] A. Garg, P. Chaturved and P. Gupta, "A review of the systemic adverse effects of areca nut or betel nut," *Indian J. Med Paediatr Oncol,* vol. 35(1), p. 3–9, Jan 2014.

[37] National Institute on Drug Abuse, "Overdose death rates," *NIH Bulletin,* Jun 2017.

[38] M. Makary, "The NFL's pink publicity stunt," *Wall St. J,* 1 Oct 2016.

[39] R. Woodford, "Lemming Suicide Myth Disney Film Faked Bogus Behavior," *Alaska Fish & Wildlife News,* September 2003.

[40] D. Dalke, *Personal Communication,* 2007.

[41] J. Avorn, "Dangerous deception — hiding the evidence of adverse drug effects," *N. Engl. J. Med.,* vol. 355, p. 21, 2006.

[42] P. Rogers, "Switching wines: rationale of methodist churches in changing a Christian tradition," Nashville, Nov 2013.

[43] E. Jewett and E. Jewett, The two wine theory: discussed by two hundred and eighty six clergymen on the basis of communion wine, New York: E. Steiger, 1888.

[44] The Holy Bible: Matthew 26.

[45] S. Hamilton, "Tirosh and Gleukos," *Battle Creek C.O.C. Bulletin,* p. 564, 4 Jul 2013.

[46] *USA Today,* p. D2, 25 May 2011.

[47] *Mayo Clinic Health Letter,* pp. 25-28, 2007.

[48] WHO, Global status report on alcohol and health, 2014, p. 7.

[49] *CDC Bulletin,* Oct 2017.

[50] *Nat'l Inst on Alcohol Abuse Bulletin,* no. 38, Oct 1997.

[51] D. Brookoff, K. O'Brien and et al, "Characteristics of participants in domestic violence," *JAMA,* vol. 277, no. 17, pp. 1369-1373, 1997.

[52] National Drug Intelligence Center, "Khat Fast Facts," [Online]. Available: www.justice.gov/archive/ndic/pubs31/31482/.

[53] M. Greener, "Drug safety on trial," *EMBO Rep,* vol. 6, p. 202–204, 2005.

[54] M. Schuckit, "Alcohol and Alcoholism," in *Harrison's Principles of Internal Medicine*, 19 ed., New York, 2015, pp. 2723-2728.

[55] Lange, Current Medical Diagnosis and Treatment, 56 ed., New York, 2017, p. 737.

[56] Diagnostic and Statistical Manual of Mental Disorders, 5th ed., Arlington VA: American Psychiatric Assn, 2013, p. 493.

[57] WHO, Global status report on alcohol and health, 2014, p. 170.

[58] *CDC Bulletin,* Feb 2018.

[59] K. Kelland, "Gates and Bloomberg create $4 million fund to fight big tobacco," *Health News,* 18 Mar 2015.

[60] "HIV Surveillance Report," CDC Center for Disease Control and Prevention Bulletin, Jun 2017.

[61] F. Bruno, "The drug problem we ignore," *The Week,* 2 Mar 2012.

[62] "Alcohol use and health," CDC Fact Sheet, Oct 2016.

[63] R. Brewer, "Reducing alcohol outlet density can reduce violent crime," CDC Bulletin, 28 May 2015.

[64] C. Campbell, R. Hahn, R. Elder and et al, "The effectiveness of limiting outlet density as a means of reducing excessive alcohol consumption and alcohol−related harms," *Am J Prev Med,* vol. 37 (6), p. 556−569, 2009.

[65] A. Lillie, *Personal Communication,* 2017.

[66] E. Hozempa, *Personal Communication,* 2017.

[67] M. Twain.

[68] W. van den Brink, "Ranking of drugs: a more balanced risk−assessment," *Lancet,* vol. 376, no. 9752, pp. 1524-1526, 6 Nov 2010.

[69] D. J. Graham, "Testimony before the US Senate," in *MPH,* Washington, DC, 18 Nov 2004.

Subject Index

Culture

Social Alcohol

Social Alcohol